PENGUIN BOOKS
THE PAIN HANDBOOK

Dr Rajat Chauhan is a student of running and pain. He is also an advocate of the GOYA (Get Off Your Arse) 'move-mint'. He has been running for over thirty-two years. After his MBBS, he went on to do sports-exercise medicine (Queen's Medical Centre, Nottingham) and osteopathy/musculoskeletal medicine (London College of Osteopathic Medicine). He has special interest in conservative management of back and knee pain. Besides heading Back 2 Fitness, a sports-medicine and musculoskeletal-medicine clinic, for the last eight years, he has been organizing the La Ultra–The High, a 333-km run in Leh-Ladakh, India, for the last seven years. He is also a contributor to several national publications (*Mint*, *Hindustan Times*, *Forbes India*, *The Hindu* and Foundingfuel.com), and a principal advisor to Adidas India.

Twitter: @drrajatchauhan
Websites: www.drrajatchauhan.com
www.thepainhandbook.com

THE PAIN HAND BOOK

A Non-Surgical Way to Manage Back, Neck and Knee Pain

Dr Rajat Chauhan

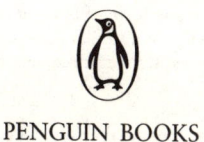

PENGUIN BOOKS

PENGUIN BOOKS

USA | Canada | UK | Ireland | Australia
New Zealand | India | South Africa | China

Penguin Books is part of the Penguin Random House group of companies whose addresses can be found at global.penguinrandomhouse.com

Published by Penguin Random House India Pvt. Ltd
7th Floor, Infinity Tower C, DLF Cyber City,
Gurgaon 122 002, Haryana, India

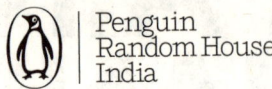

First published in Penguin Books by Penguin Random House India 2016

Text and Illustrations copyright © Rajat Chauhan 2016
Page 301 is an extension of the copyright page
Illustrations by Jemastock and Adimas

All rights reserved

10 9 8 7 6 5 4 3 2 1

The views and opinions expressed in this book are the author's own and the facts are as reported by him which have been verified to the extent possible, and the publishers are not in any way liable for the same.

ISBN 9780143420118

Typeset in Sabon by Manipal Digital Systems, Manipal
Printed at Thomson Press India Ltd, New Delhi

This book is sold subject to the condition that it shall not, by way of trade or otherwise, be lent, resold, hired out, or otherwise circulated without the publisher's prior consent in any form of binding or cover other than that in which it is published and without a similar condition including this condition being imposed on the subsequent purchaser.

www.penguinbooksindia.com

Hi Rajat,

I am not so well these days. The cancer (breast) has got the better of me and has finally won. I have very little time, weeks perhaps. I am under hospice care now and just live one day at a time. It's not how I thought things would be so make sure you enjoy every day.

Big hugs to you, my 'student'.

X Anne

Anne passed away on Monday, 27 June 2016. This one is for you—the one who held my unconfident, unsure hand, and taught me all about 'the touch'. The one who taught me how to 'feel' and 'treat the patient' not with my hands alone but with my heart, too. It is an art that is lost in today's instant gratification healthcare industry where a patient is just a number.

I also dedicate this book to all those who have suffered and will suffer from pain in the future. Take care of yourself. You are very special.

CONTENTS

Foreword ix
Modern Version of the Hippocratic Oath xi
Prologue: Why Me? xiii

1. Why You Need This Book 1
2. Getting to Know Yourself 18
3. What You Should Do When You Have Back Pain 51
4. Tests and Investigations 79
5. Common Diagnosis: Causes of Back Pain 93
6. Proactively Managing Back Pain 105
7. The Three Musketeers: Foot (and Ankle), Knee and Hip (FKH) 158
8. Other Common Aches and Pains 201
9. Pain Is Inevitable, Suffering Is Optional 213

Acknowledgements 285
Notes 289

FOREWORD

The back is a complex structure made of multiple bones separated by discs and held together by strong ligaments and muscles. It is designed to provide flexibility in all directions through facet joints while protecting the spinal cord within it and nerves exiting through the neural foramina at each level. Each of its components is a possible source of pain which can be acute or chronic, of differing severity and sometimes associated with neurological deficit such as weakness, numbness or bladder/bowel incompetence. Unfortunately, treatment today is based on Magnetic Resonance Imagings (MRIs), which, though extremely useful in eliminating serious disorders such as tumours, trauma and infections such as tuberculosis, are of little value in the common causes associated with day-to-day strain such as disc pain or age-related degeneration. Most of these can be managed conservatively by a good chiropractor or physiotherapist under the guidance of an orthopaedic surgeon to avoid complications. Unfortunately, the tool which revolutionized diagnosis of the back is now being used to scare unsuspecting patients into surgery without informing them of the complications. This is often more disabling than the original problem especially in the elderly. Keep an eye on your back—knife-happy surgeons are waiting to literally stab you in the back!

15 September 2016 Dr (Brig.) B.K. Singh,
Gurgaon joint replacement surgeon,
founder of the joint
replacement centre at
Army R & R Hospital, Delhi.

MODERN VERSION OF THE HIPPOCRATIC OATH

I swear to fulfil, to the best of my ability and judgement, this covenant . . .

I will respect the hard-won scientific gains of those physicians in whose steps I walk, and gladly share such knowledge as is mine with those who are to follow.

I will apply, for the benefit of the sick, all measures which are required, avoiding those twin traps of over-treatment and therapeutic nihilism.

I will remember that there is art to medicine as well as science, and that warmth, sympathy and understanding may outweigh the surgeon's knife or the chemist's drug.

I will not be ashamed to say 'I know not', nor will I fail to call in my colleagues when the skills of another are needed for a patient's recovery.

I will respect the privacy of my patients, for their problems are not disclosed to me so that the world may know. Most especially must I tread with care in matters of life and death. Above all, I must not play God.

I will remember that I do not treat a fever chart, a cancerous growth, but a sick human being, whose illness may affect the person's family and economic stability. My responsibility includes these related problems, if I am to care adequately for the sick.

I will prevent disease whenever I can, for prevention is preferable to cure.

I will remember that I remain a member of society, with special obligations to all my fellow human beings, those sound of mind and body as well as the infirm.

If I do not violate this oath, may I enjoy life and art, respected while I live and remembered with affection thereafter. May I always act so as to preserve the finest traditions of my calling and may I long experience the joy of healing those who seek my help.

—Written in 1964 by Louis Lasagna, Academic Dean of the School of Medicine at Tufts University, and used in many medical schools today.

PROLOGUE: WHY ME?

Death does not concern us, because as long as we exist, death is not here.
And when it does come, we no longer exist.

—Epicurus

A long time ago, before we were born, we ran as sperms towards the ovum. What happened after that? Since then, why have we all become such slobs and gone against the basic rule of nature? We moved to be born. We need to keep moving to stay alive; else we'll merely exist.

I am one of you. I have been living with pain for more than two decades now. For more than a decade I have had a couple of cervical (neck) disc bulges, which occasionally cause pain down my left hand, and a couple of disc bulges in the lumbar spine (lower back), which cause weakness and pain down my left leg. Besides that, I have a meniscus injury in my right knee that has been causing pain, off and on, for over two decades now. Most of 2015 and 2016 was emotionally tough for me. I pretty much hit rock bottom. I had to dig in deep to bounce back to normal life—seeing patients with pain, helping runners reach levels they thought they were not capable of, writing on a regular basis, and catering to all kinds of sports needs of students at Ashoka University in Sonepat, Haryana, an institution which is truly world class in liberal arts. I also put together the sixth edition of La Ultra—The High, a 333-km run held in Leh-Ladakh, which crosses three of the highest motorable mountain passes. As I am the founder and race director, I had to stay calm and not show my feelings because other people trusted me with their lives.

It is very easy to give up on life. I've been fortunate to have been guided by the very best on how to carry on with life—running being the most important of them all. That's exactly why I call myself a student of running and pain, for life. It's a never-ending journey, and when it finally does get over, it doesn't bother us any more.

I am an ultra-marathoner, i.e., someone who runs more than a marathon distance (42.195 km) on a regular basis. I am also a medical osteopath, a physician of musculoskeletal medicine (equivalent to an orthopaedic surgeon minus the surgery) and sports-exercise medicine (someone not only interested in treating sports injuries, or preventing injuries but using exercise as a modality to treat disease and pain). I like to call myself advocate of GOYA (Get Off Your Arse). I run a chain of medical clinics that take up more than 8 hours of my day. I also love writing columns and blogs on running and pain. I have also been doing a weekly running podcast, Move-Mint, for *Mint*, a business newspaper. Basically, I live my life the way I want. And if I can, you can too.

I first got to know pain at a wholly different level at the age of nine when I was introduced to running at Wynberg Allen School in Mussoorie, located at the foothills of the Himalayas. At the age of ten, it wasn't simply about getting to the finishing line. Our sports teacher Champa Dhakpa, would happily cane the kid who came last. His thought process was simple and straightforward, 'If you can do more, why be content with less?' Hence, all of us tried our best to not come last. I am very thankful to Champa Sir, who in his own way instilled in all of us the determination to keep pushing our comfort zone, because that's where the real change happens.

We were forced to run fast to avoid one kind of pain, obviously putting our body through another kind of pain. On weekends, the top six finishers would get a mango drink. Some of the kids were naturally gifted, but I had to struggle. I started putting my body through more pain during each run, so I could finish sixth or fifth on weekends. There was no incentive to push harder or finish at a higher position, as there were no extra points or mango drinks for that.

The pain I talk about above is not the kind that needed medical attention, but it made me stronger. All sportspersons train to push their bodies harder. They just grind their teeth and keep going. This actually makes them better at tolerating pain in life, apart from becoming better athletes. This helps increase both their pain threshold (the point at which you complain of pain) and pain tolerance (how long you're willing to endure a given level of pain). Newer studies[1] state that getting fitter doesn't improve your pain tolerance, but repeatedly enduring pain changes your perception of it. You end up training your mind as well as your muscles.

By the time I was seventeen, I had run a half-marathon (21 km) in one hour and eighteen minutes. Running taught me how to respect pain and fatigue. It was something to listen to and work around. I could push my body a lot more. Once the realization comes that pain is only a messenger, it helps you perform a lot better. Not only running, but climbing stairs, lifting your grandson, sitting properly, walking, going on a date, making the date more colourful and having sex, watching a three-hour movie, taking long flights, scuba-diving and bungee jumping can all be done with greater facility if we realize this truth.

When I run for long distances and there is pain, I start listening to it: 'I am pain. I've been around for as long as humanity has been. For ages, I have been given a bad reputation, making me sound as if I am the enemy. When, in fact, my intentions are good. My interest is your well-being. I'm simply a messenger. Once you start understanding my messages and act on them appropriately, you will go into a Zen-like zone. Nothing will ever bother you again.'

Also, it has been repeatedly mentioned in peer-reviewed medical journals that to understand and address pain, one needs to have the knowledge of almost all the fields that deal with pain. I am fortunate enough to be one of the rare doctors in India with that distinction. I wouldn't dare say that I know it all, but I do try to learn about any field that addresses back pain, whether it is traditional or alternative medicine. I have been requested twice (2014 and 2015) by the *Hindustan Times* to contribute to the HT Leadership Summit series by talking about 'How to Get India to Be a Fitter Nation'. From mid-2014 to mid-2016, I was the director of sports-exercise at Ashoka University, where I used to see a lot of students between the ages of 17 and 25 with back, neck and knee pain. Earlier this would happen three to four decades later in their lives. It's the modern sedentary lifestyle that's to be blamed.

Through this book, I will introduce you to the holistic approach of understanding and managing pain like never before, with the intent to empower you with the knowledge. It'll not be a passive approach where you end up being a helpless spectator, which is the case today. You will be in control. That means that you'll have to be proactively involved. It's you who has the pain. It's your problem. Outsourcing it isn't going to make a long-term difference. You will not be at the mercy of the so-called experts. That's my simple philosophy to address your pain—to make you better informed. I want you to know the simple, key things that completely changed my outlook on pain during my education.

I have been fortunate to have been mentored by some eminent and experienced doctors, therapists and scientists from different fields like anaesthesiology, orthopaedics, rheumatology, osteopathy, physiotherapy, psychology, and so on, who had a special interest in pain. The best part is that they came from different countries with diverse cultures, such as the UK, Australia, the US, Canada, France, South Africa, Germany, Finland, Iran and Greece. This has given me a comprehensive overview of pain.

After having interacted and trained with all these specialists from different backgrounds, I found that the one thing that differentiated them from other top-notch doctors and therapists was that they were always looking at a proactive solution for the person in pain, unlike a passive treatment prescribed by most other doctors. The people I trained under wanted patients to move. They wanted patients to think. They wanted patients to be in control.

In 1994, I developed a retinal detachment in my right eye, which could have led to blindness. I was in my first year of MBBS then and only eighteen years old. When I asked the surgeon, who operated on me, how soon I could get back to running, he looked puzzled. 'Are you planning on going to the Olympics? If not, why do you want to run?' That was like a death sentence for me. Had he told me before operating, there was a good chance that I would have opted for lifelong running rather than saving my sight. Running was, and is, my life. It's never judged me. It is right beside me all the time, just waiting for me. Even though I was just starting my education to be a doctor, I had already started disliking medicine and was almost on the verge of hating it. I found the people judgemental, as they took decisions on behalf of patients on how they should lead their lives. However, I did listen to my surgeon for a bit.

The only lecture I remember from medical school is a guest lecture. It was by Dr B. M. Hegde, an eminent cardiologist and former vice chancellor of Manipal University. He spoke about how amazing our body was and that it could heal itself in the right environment. These words have stayed with me since then.

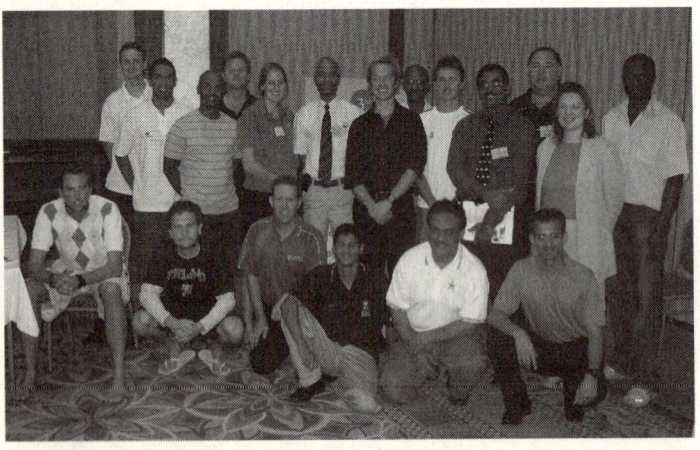

Dr Rajat Chauhan (extreme right, sitting) at the third World Congress of Science and Medicine in Cricket held in the Caribbean in 2007.

It wasn't until 2002 that I decided to start running again. I was doing my masters in sports-exercise medicine at Queen's Medical Centre at the University of Nottingham at that time. Here I was fortunate to have Dr Peter L. Gregory, then the chief medical officer of England and Wales Cricket Board, and the course director of the postgraduate programme in sports-exercise medicine, as my immediate supervisor. He has been an amazing guide since then. It's such amazing human beings who teach you more about life—lessons that are not written in books. That's what makes one a better doctor. It's not simply about how good a technician you are.

He told me that if he could go back in time, he would learn how to use his hands better to treat sportspersons and other patients. He was instrumental in directing me towards London College of Osteopathic Medicine (LCOM), which really changed my approach to medicine. It would be incorrect to mention only one or two tutors from this institute, as all of them were amazing. However, Dr Roderic Macdonald (the then principal of LCOM and the president of British Institute of Musculoskeletal Medicine) and Anne Gibbons (professor, medical osteopathy) were the ones who taught me a lot more than what osteopathic medicine could alone.

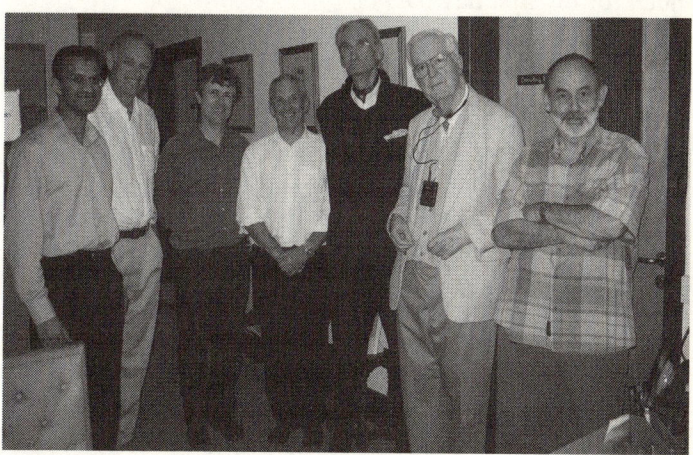

During a workshop conducted by Dr Rajat Chauhan's tutors and senior colleagues in 2004. (From left to right) Dr Rajat Chauhan, Dr Mike Hopkins, Dr Peter Wilkin, Dr Michael Monk, Dr Mike Burleigh Carson, Dr Douglas Longden and Dr Roderic Macdonald.

I thought I had learnt all there was to learn about pain from ancient and new books alike, but my tutors and mentors in the two fields introduced me to pain like never before. After I graduated from LCOM, some of us would get together for masterclass workshops, where I would be the youngest, at least by three decades if not more.

At Nottingham, I signed up for the university's running club and joined the 'kids' who were almost a decade younger to me for a 'short' 8-km run. I had broken the cardinal rule of exercising or running. If you have taken a long break, you always start from scratch and never bank on your past laurels. You constantly build on them and carry on from there. Not even halfway into the run, every possible muscle in my body started hurting as the students were way too fast for me to keep up with and that distance was just a bit too much for my first day back.

It was as ironical as it could get. There I was, at one of the top sports-exercise medicine institutes in the world, trying to learn how to take care of sports injuries, but I didn't know how to tackle my own. Severe shin pain persisted after just that first overenthusiastic run. It hurt to walk. Luckily for me, a top track and field doctor was taking guest lectures at the time. When asked for help, he gave me some tips, but nothing changed. It took me a couple of months of being a slob to get better.

I picked up ultra-running when I moved to London in 2003 to do medical osteopathy. The first multistage ultra I attempted was from Paris to London. I covered the distance of a marathon (42.195 km) or more (60 km daily) for eight consecutive days. On the second day of this run, I developed some pain just above the left ankle. A member of the support staff for the run applied cold spray on it. She sprayed too much, too close, burning my skin. It was only a muscular strain to begin with, but now I couldn't even touch it, forget massaging it. Next morning,

I couldn't even stand on the leg, so I left an hour before the others, and managed to finish the day's distance.

On the fourth day, the pain was phenomenal. Again, I left earlier than the rest, limping my way through. The same staff member, who had sprayed my leg, feeling guilty, joined me on the bike for the first 20 km. She then started pacing me. Incidentally, she herself is a decent triathlete. She pushed me hard to run the last 10 km of the 60 km that day in forty-two minutes. For the non-runners amongst you, that's decently fast, even by itself. On the fifth day, my foot was so swollen that it wouldn't even fit into the shoe, so I decided to take off the laces and use crepe bandage to wrap around the shoe. I had to limp sideways and at times backwards to move forward. Yes, it was tricky. I moved at a snail's pace. Now I couldn't even bear weight on the left leg. Even though I had to quit at the end of the day, I learnt how to manage pain and carry on.

There is always more to learn. Throughout, I have managed pain, giving it the respect it demands. In return, the pain has let me pass as well. It has helped me raise my pain tolerance and pain threshold.

Professor Timothy Noakes[2], an authority on sports medicine and science, in his thought-provoking book *Challenging Beliefs: Memoirs of a Career*, makes some interesting observations that resonate with my own thoughts. His teachers also taught him that exercise was dangerous for human health. Since he felt better after exercising, he concluded that authority and conventional wisdom wasn't to be trusted. Probably that's what led me to follow his work closely, even though I had attended only a handful of his lectures at various international sports medicine conferences in London and Cape Town.

He acknowledges in his book that it's only during exercise that we access parts of the brain that normally remain untouched. We become more aware of our bodies, and recognize that we truly don't know the limits, which are far beyond anything we ever thought.

It might sound ironical, but in 2008, just a week before the launch of Back 2 Fitness, my clinic that focuses on pain management and sports-exercise medicine, I experienced severe neck pain. On clinical examination and investigation, it was confirmed to be caused by two irritated cervical nerves because of disc herniation at corresponding levels. This was leading to severe pain, numbness and a pins-and-needle sensation down my left arm.

A few years before that, while doing musculoskeletal training in London, I had severe lower back pain, which was supposedly coming from two lumbar disc bulges. I also happen to have a right knee injury (meniscal tear). But I have learnt, over the years, not to let that interfere with the quality of my life. I am a firm believer in the following: If you are not running (living) on the edge, you are wasting too much space. Effectively, I like to push my body but with respect. I can run 100 km in under 10 hours, I have run a marathon distance (42 km) on five consecutive days a few times now and have run a half-marathon distance (21 km) on every day of the month on a few occasions now.

I also started La Ultra—The High[3] in 2010, initially 222 km distance, which even the adventure wing of the Indian Army, top medical doctors and locals of the area pronounced impossible. This event pushes the boundaries of what we consider to be humanly impossible. I believe we don't know those limits yet. I like to call it the ultra marathon because we attempt to convert a dangerous run into a difficult one. Since too many participants were able to finish 222 km, I have now increased the distance to 333 km. One has to cross three mountain passes, at times run at altitudes which are almost half as high as what jets fly at, all to be covered in three days (72 hours).

Pain is similar to the high Himalayan mountains. If you plan to defeat them, they will crush you whenever they feel like, but if you respect them, the mammoth mountains will suddenly become gentle and let you enjoy the beauty and cross the boundaries that you thought impossible. Participants coming to my race in Leh have demonstrated that time and again.

This doesn't only apply to doing crazy activities, but also living with pain and managing it well in daily life, doing regular chores. We just have been playing too safe, a bit too much, for way too long. My doctor colleagues almost recommend lying down for life, since moving hurts, without realizing that we were actually made to move.

In 2013, I trained eighteen women from all walks of life, ranging from thirteen to sixty years of age, for a 'zero to 6 km' running programme. It taught me something fundamental. Doing anything from nothing is a lot more difficult than doing more, even if it is extremely daunting. All these women had attempted various training programmes in the past but had not been able to carry on for long. It made me realize that all of us are fighting our own battles day in and day out. There are challenges and there will always be challenges. It's easy to call it quits. We need to take pain head-on rather than shying away. The women surprised themselves by doing a lot more than what they had thought themselves capable of doing.

I am not suggesting you run 100 km, or take part in the insane La Ultra—The High in Leh-Ladakh, but you need to reclaim your life and do justice to it. For this, you need to understand your body and pain. You'll be surprised to learn that you simply don't need to live with it, even though my doctor colleagues' advice might sound like a death sentence to you.

I have experienced pain when pushing the body to perform better while running, but I have also experienced agonizing pain in the neck and back on a regular basis.

Contrary to popular belief, once I started appreciating pain it pretty much showed me the way. It let me move and even run again. My running helped me understand my body better than my medical degrees did. I listen better to my body but I am always looking to push that much harder, as only then can I become stronger and better at managing pain.

As professor Noakes observes, the diseased, who become athletes (physically more active), have had a great influence on medicine: they have taught us (doctors) that there is a healthy way to be ill.

It's a fact that individuals who have had back pain are at a higher risk of getting another episode as opposed to someone who has never had back pain. But if you decide to be in control and be more physically active, it evens out. You actually get to a stronger position than the slob who hasn't had back pain yet. For him or her, it's a ticking time bomb.

If you experience pain while moving and doing regular chores, you might become too apprehensive to continue doing them. However, it is a catch-22 situation. If you don't

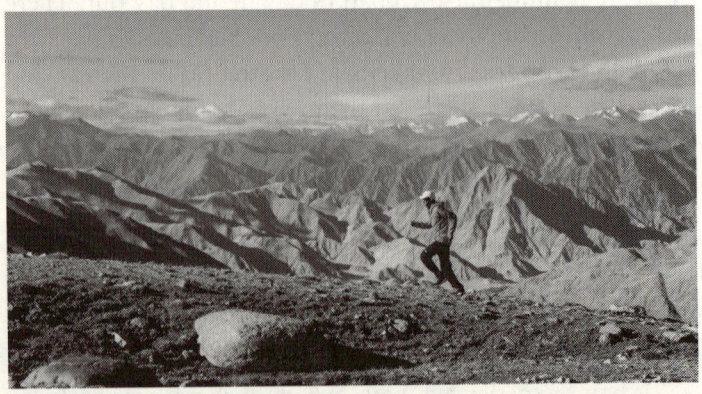

Dr Rajat Chauhan running up Wari La in Leh-Ladakh during the 2016 edition of La Ultra—The High

move, it'll only hurt more when you do try to move. We need to appreciate that simple movements are not going to make your condition worse. Your pain is out of proportion to how serious your condition is. The fear of pain is worse than the actual pain itself.

Even on days when the pain is really bad, it is strongly recommended that you be as mobile as possible. If the pain persists over the years, you could have days of pain on a regular basis. You need to move. Once you move and exercise, your muscles will become more independent. Rather than being a load on the body, they will actually support your body. Along with improving pain tolerance and pain threshold, it'll help the largest system in your body, the musculoskeletal system, to work more efficiently.

The amount and intensity with which you move around could vary depending on your pain. I completely appreciate that this is easier said than done, but you need to get more in control.

Even on the worst days, if nothing else, you need to do your breathing exercises and meditation throughout the day. When there is pain, all of us have a tendency to stiffen up. This could be helpful over shorter durations, but over longer periods it is counterproductive and will only make your pain worse. When you breathe easy and meditate, the intention is to let go of pain and not tense your body. More about this is discussed in the book.

Keep miling and smiling.

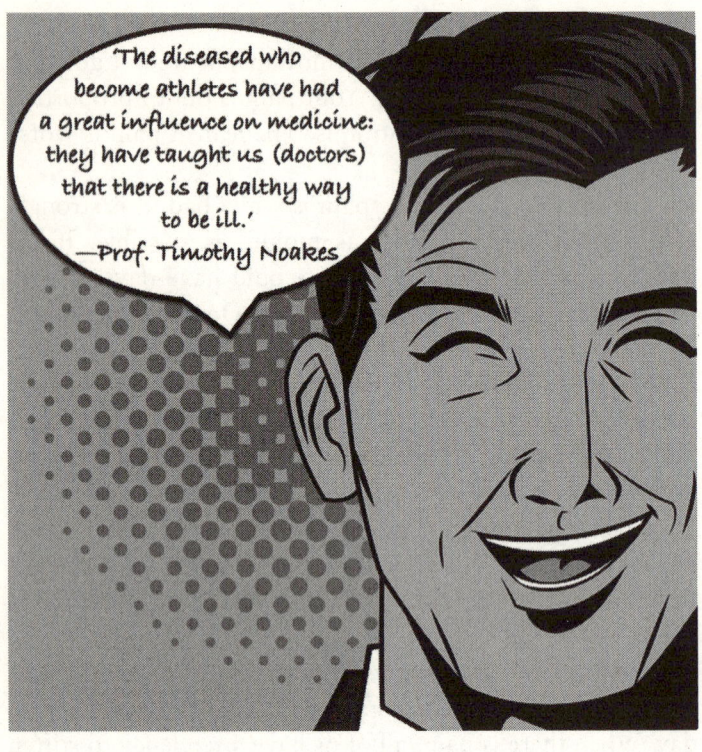

1

WHY YOU NEED THIS BOOK

It's important to clarify at the very outset that this book does not intend to replace medical advice or be a textbook on pain. The purpose of this book is to make the sufferer more aware about the body, without going into too many technicalities. The main focus of this book is on what you can do for yourself rather than highlight details of all the medical and surgical treatments available.

Why a Book on Back (Neck, Knee and Hip) Pain?

Pain in the back and neck is by far the number one reason for Indians (and others too, worldwide) for the 'years of life lived with disability'.[1]

It then might come as a surprise to you that medicine textbooks, such as Davidson's *Principles and Practice of Medicine*, which are referred by medical students in colleges, have less than two pages on back and neck pain—the most commonly experienced pain.

Back and neck pain might not kill you, but it won't let you live either. It's like being madly in love with someone but not being able to be with that person.

Depressive disorders come a close second. The tricky part is that there is a major overlap between back and neck pain and depression. It's like a vicious circle. They almost feed off each other. And the fact that a lot of people suffer from it, shows that modern lifestyle is a bane of human society. To address it, we can't have the oversimplified, unidirectional cause-and-effect model that has been suggested for ages now. For once, modern Western medicine has failed the society. Or has it?

Back, neck and knee pain takes its toll not only on the individual suffering from it, but also on the family, workplace and society. An increased incidence of back pain makes doctors of any speciality advise on it without having a solid basic foundation. The tremendous amount of misinformation makes the situation worse.

Not surprisingly then, my healthcare colleagues the world over, including the 'experts' in the field, have been addressing these pains with a simple model—an injury to bones, vertebrae, muscles, ligaments, tendons, fascia and so on causes the pain. When, as a matter of fact, it is the brain that decides to cause pain, and it's finally *you* who suffers.

If there is one solution to this problem, it is to be better informed. Hence this book.

Play a Proactive Role in Solving Your Problem

You need this book because you or your loved ones are suffering from pain. Stop outsourcing your problems. You need to solve them yourself. I will help you do it, but you have to participate proactively. Else, you won't be able to rid yourself of it. Even if you do, it will soon come back looking for you. Possibly, with a vengeance.

It's your job to be better informed rather than blaming the 'experts' years later.

This book is not about voodoo or magic to relieve you of back pain. It's an evidence-based approach, based on recent medical research and guidelines, recommended by leading institutions globally. Even though experts would know what worked in most of the cases, it is you who knows the nature of *your* pain. We together need to figure out what will work in your case. Some would say it's guesswork; I would call it 'informed guesswork' that will get you back on your feet.

Pain, experienced by almost everyone at some point in their lives in varying degrees, is an exceedingly complicated phenomenon. If cancer is called the 'emperor of all maladies', back pain might well be the empress. It'll make your life miserable. The societal cost of back pain is three times higher than the total cost of all types of cancers.[2] Lower back pain affects up to 80 per cent of people at some point in their life, and neck pain affects up to 50 per cent of the population.[3] These numbers have risen tremendously in the last two decades courtesy drastic changes in our lifestyles. The good news is that most people get cured without surgical intervention. Even among those who suffer pain longer than expected, the majority don't need any surgeries.

The most common perception is that disc bulge and rupture are the biggest reasons for lower back pain, but that's not true. Doctors need to look at muscle tension and spasm, laxity of ligaments, muscle imbalance, joint instability, etc., which can't be examined with gadgets. Only doctors trained in 'touch' and 'palpation' can find out the reason for the pain. Sadly, today's medical colleges don't cover that either. They emphasize on high-tech investigative tools and recommend drugs or surgeries. At times they treat patients via electronic communication, even without meeting them in person.

Case: P.P. Pande, seventy-seven years old

Pande visited us in July 2012 with a complaint of poor mobility and pain in joints. He had been suffering from ankylosing spondylitis for over a decade. He wanted to get cured of the pain and have better mobility.

Ankylosing spondylitis leads the vertebrae in the spine to fuse together, reducing the flexibility of the spine. It eventually leads to a hunched forward posture. When the upper and mid-back gets involved, ribs have reduced movement too. This causes difficulty in breathing. However, the healthcare industry doesn't have much to offer. One thing that is completely overlooked is that as a result of the stiffness, the patient starts moving less; this further leads to joints not being able to move freely. That's a domino effect right there.

The best of medical literature out there says that there is no cure for ankylosing spondylitis. Leave a patient with that thought and what do you expect? I am not suggesting we need to lie. However, we do need to tell the patient the whole story—the story that even we didn't know till very recently. It needs to be emphasized that the simplest of activities like breathing will become difficult. It's important that they exercise their joints more often. By doing this, the domino effect can be reversed into a positive. Strength training can play an important role in achieving this.

The movement of Pande's spine (neck, upper back and lower back) and bigger joints (hips, knees and shoulders) was severely restricted. His ribs too didn't have enough movement, restricting the expansion of his lungs. There was muscle wasting throughout the body. His symptoms were classic textbook ones for advanced ankylosing spondylitis.

Given his age, most doctors gave up. Probably that was the reason why he wasn't excited about visiting doctors since they really weren't his friends.

It was important to first boost his self-confidence and assure him that he would be mobile again, since in the last few years he had been physically inactive. He had simply given up on himself. The treatment was designed to improve the range of movement of his joints and mobility (keeping in mind that he used to tire easily). So, various breathing exercises were given along with the spine mobility programme. More importantly, he was encouraged to believe in himself. It had to be made clear to him that it just wasn't a false hope that we were working on.

In a case like this, pacing is very important. You never give too much too soon. Go slow. Go at just the right pace. Too little could also mean wasting too much time. He was started on daily short walks to improve his cardiorespiratory fitness. Simultaneously, he was put on a strength-training programme that focused on his core—hip, knee and upper body.

He also underwent a few sessions of dry needling (medical acupuncture) when there was a severe tightness/tenderness around his right hip. It eased the muscles immediately and the pain was reduced.

Pande was initially resistant to the sudden change in his activity levels but he was persistent and showed perseverance to the solution offered to him.

Within six months, Pande was regularly going for his evening walks. Now, he was not bogged down with the inabilities of his own body. Instead, he made sure that he was physically more active in order to reduce his symptoms of aches and pains.

He is now eighty and free of painkillers, is more mobile and flexible and enjoys going for walks. He does not need anybody to support him in his day-to-day activities. His quality of life has improved.

Testimonials

P. P. Pande

'Back 2 Fitness'! Such an apt name. In July 2012, I hobbled into the establishment with a body full of sick bones and sinews, and a mind almost resigned to a life of an invalid. I was up and about in about six months after just an hour-long session, twice a week, which later came down to once a week.

Many thanks to Dr Chauhan and his very competent team of therapists, I'm now free of my aches and pains and especially of painkillers.

Mahima, P. P. Pande's Daughter

I would also like to add my personal note of thanks to the team at Back 2 Fitness for making the journey for my father from painful to pain-free such a wonderful one. The level of individual attention, patience and belief that they've shown has gone a long way in making him a healthier and a happier person.

The reason why the treatment and management of pain are not where they should be is as complicated as the subject itself. Also, the age at which people suffer with neck and back pains has reduced markedly. Earlier, back and neck pains used to happen in the fifth and sixth decade. In my own practice, I frequently come across patients with severe neck and back pain. It is common in working professionals in their twenties and thirties, and even in children as young as ten! It's a consequence of the way we live now.

The most commonly prescribed solutions are either painkillers or surgery. Other than in acute pain, the role of painkillers is very questionable. Most painkillers only mask the superficial symptoms, that too temporarily. In any case, long-term consumption of anti-inflammatory drugs is not advisable.

Even though surgery might seem like the only way to address the underlying problem, it really isn't. If all goes well, which most surgeons are competent enough of achieving, what is addressed is the effect and not the cause. Plus, very rarely do surgeons play a role in patient management, post-surgery. Even if the best material is put in, and the 'source' of pain is removed, it will soon come back. To solve this, we need to address you as human beings, not just as 'painful backs'. My intention is not to say that medicine or surgery is entirely useless, or that other doctors are incompetent. My only point, which will echo throughout this book, is that treating back pain is both an individualistic and holistic venture and it cannot be done in any other way.

History of Pain and Challenging Its 'Beliefs'

Pain is inevitable, suffering is optional.

—Buddha

As mentioned earlier, there is too much misinformation out there about pain, especially back pain. It's rightly said that in India every one is a consultant. Pain happens to be one such field that everyone specializes in, or at least that's what they think. Advisors range from your parents, accountant, cobbler, driver, cook, lawyer, plumber to qualified doctors. But good advice is hard to come by, whether from doctors or your family and friends. All of them have good intentions, but most of the times it ends up making your pain worse.

The simple fact is, you don't have to suffer with this pain. It's your choice, but for that you need to take control. You need to be better informed about pain.

Definition of Pain

'Pain is an unpleasant sensory and *emotional* experience associated with actual or *potential* tissue damage, or *described* in terms of such damage' —updated definition of pain by The International Association for the Study of Pain (IASP).

Focus on the words 'emotional', 'potential' and 'described'. Did you know or were you explained the role these play by your treating doctor or physiotherapist? Emotional experience is almost never addressed by the current conventional medical model even though it plays a major role. How about potential tissue damage? This refers to no real injury but one that could have happened. The more patients reach out to Dr Google, the more they will know about the described symptoms in their condition and soon enough they will start showing those symptoms, without having a 'real' injury. Most colleagues would say that such patients are faking their symptoms or are malingerers.

When we read any of the above definitions of pain, we somehow are not able to relate to it. It feels like something that would never happen to us and it is just an alien terminology.

On the other hand, the Merriam-Webster English dictionary defines pain as 'a state of physical, emotional, or mental lack of well-being or physical, emotional, or mental uneasiness that ranges from mild discomfort or dull distress to acute often unbearable agony, may be generalized or localized, and is the consequence of being injured or hurt physically or mentally or of some derangement of or lack of equilibrium in the physical or mental functions (as through disease), and that usually produces a reaction of wanting to avoid, escape, or destroy the causative factor and its effects'.

It's a long definition, but is in simple language. Like the intention of my work, it's simplifying things that I am decent at, whether it be terminology or advice.

> The goal wasn't to make patients better; it was to make patients feel better. Pain is the most complex human experience. That it involves your past life, your current life, your interactions, your family.
>
> —Dr John J. Bonica, founding father of the study of pain management.

Dr John J. Bonica, known as the founding father of the study of pain management, arrived at this conclusion as early as the 1950s. He believed that to achieve this, your past life, your current life, your interactions, your family had to be involved.

Bonica was also a professional wrestler and saw pain from close quarters. He felt it. He lived it. And it made it impossible for him to ignore it in others. Out of that empathy, he spun a whole new field, played a major role in getting medicine to acknowledge pain.

The intent of this book is similar to what Dr Bonica did. This book will focus primarily on back pain (and knee pain) as pain is too vast a subject.

History of Back Pain and Its Knowledge: Questioning Conventional Wisdom in Back Pain Treatment

Back pain has probably existed from the time Homo sapiens decided to go against nature, i.e., gravity, and stand upright. The resultant disability is a more recent phenomenon.

Let's look at it this way: 'Pain is what the world does to you, suffering is what you do to yourself.'[4]

As Wadell[5] says, in his ground-breaking paper on back pain, 'The real question is when simple backache became what we now regard as a medical problem?'

The word 'pain' comes from *Poine* (or *Poena*), the monstrous drakaina (she-dragon), who was once summoned from the underworld by Apollo to punish mortal fools.[6] The gods had entrusted her with revenge, retribution, vengeance, punishment for murder and manslaughter.

The oldest document that describes the treatment of back pain dates back to 3,500 years ago. These papyri were buried in the Upper Nile near Thebes, Egypt. They were found by grave robbers and sold to Edwin Smith in 1862.[7] This document abruptly ends before the treatment starts. Modern medicine is based on the disease model of illness which flourished during the Renaissance. Before that, during the dark ages, back pain was thought to be due to external influences.[8]

In almost all cultures, people attribute current sufferings as punishment for misdeeds of either previous life, or even of the same one. It is fascinating then to know that Hippocrates, the father of medicine, who lived from 460 BCE to 377 BCE, almost two-and-a-half millenniums ago, didn't believe in cursed diseases and miraculous cures. On the other hand, he believed that environmental factors, including hygiene, diet and climate, have a profound influence on both the mind and the body. He also prescribed chewing willow leaves and barks for pain to women in childbirth, following in the footsteps of Egyptians who had known of this since 1500 BCE. One of the earliest forms of aspirin was actually derived from myrtle leaves, willow bark, and birch bark, which contain a pain-relieving substance called salicin.[9]

Primitive man understood pain when it was visible, like a cut or scrape, but didn't understand it as well when it was internal. Doctors in some cultures would cut a hole in the skull to let the pain out.[10] In the Middle Ages, it was believed that it was better to have more drugs to treat pain.[11] Does it not suggest that we are back in the Middle Ages as doctors write down more than a dozen different medicines on a single prescription sheet for back pain?

Up till the Industrial Revolution, especially the building of the railways, chronic back pain was not thought to be due to an injury.[12] The condition came to be known as Railway Spine as it was experienced by workers when they were laying the railway tracks.[13]

It was in the sixteenth century that Valerius Cordus and Paracelsus prepared ether by distilling sulphuric acid (oil of vitriol) with fortified wine to produce oleum vitrioli dulce (sweet oil of vitriol). Paracelsus observed that the ether caused chickens to fall asleep and awaken unharmed, but these properties were not thought to have any medical implications. It wasn't until January 1842 when William E. Clarke, a medical student from Rochester, New York, may have administered the first ether anaesthetic.[14]

In 1853, Queen Victoria was the first to be given anaesthesia for her eighth childbirth, and then again for the ninth. It was through chloroform, administered by Dr John Snow,[15] who was then criticized by *The Lancet*, a much sought-after medical journal then and today.

Nothing has really changed. Poly-pharmacy (multi-drug) approach, as in the Middle Ages, is now practised widely. We now live in an instant gratification society. Demand and supply has led to this. Today's situation cannot be attributed to just one of them. We seem to be ignoring the suffering and the emotional context, which was addressed very well in the past.[16]

Bed Rest Is Bad for Your Back: Basis for Today's Popular Approach to Back Pain[17]

Current conventional treatment offered for back pain is based on the evolution of orthopaedics as a speciality, and its key principle of rest. Even though Sydenham (1743) had insisted that arthritic patients should be kept mobile 'since keeping them on a bed constantly promotes and augments the disease', bed rest as a treatment had been proposed in modern medicine by John Hunter (1749). Bed rest became an orthopaedic principle, which hasn't changed much in practice over these years, in spite of immense amount of scientific evidence to the contrary. This really was the beginning of making patients take a passive role in their sufferings.

It was only in 1828[18] that Thomas Brown, a physician at Glasgow Royal Infirmary, suggested that the vertebral column and the nervous system could be sources of back pain. Even today, high-tech investigations like MRIs only look at the physical damage, without taking the whole patient into account; leave alone the bigger ecosystem he or she is a part of. This could be the main contributor of pain.

Hugh Owen Thomas (1843–91), who came from the long line of Welsh bone-setters, was the pioneer of modern orthopaedics in Britain. Even though he incorporated some of his skills in modern orthopaedics, he rejected many of the bone-setters' principles, especially that of mobilization. In addition, he advocated best rest—'enforced, uninterrupted and prolonged bed rest'—which is completely different from the philosophy of staying active and mobile—something recent guidelines are recommending. This was achieved by bed rest, bracing and surgical fusion.

Not all suggested prolonged rest. In one of the earliest orthopaedic texts on back pain, there is a lecture by Johnstone (1884). He advised against bed rest in chronic back pain, since he believed bed rest was a cause of back pain.

By 1900, a standard treatment offered for the back was two to six weeks of strict bed rest. Somehow, that has been so ingrained in the system that even today most doctors follow the same recommendation. Most institutions are excellent at dulling the sharpest of minds, so they wouldn't question the most ridiculous practices.

Prolonged bed rest was promoted because it was believed that the lower back pain was due to traumatic inflammation, which had to be given an opportunity to heal.

Rudolf Virchow (1821–1902), the father of modern pathology, was of the opinion that when a diagnosis is used to identify a disease, these syndromes have an underlying morbid anatomical basis awaiting demonstration. Virchow classified diseases based on anatomical sites, subdivided them into the possible pathological processes which might affect each, and tried to fit every clinical presentation into one of the classes formed. Even today, after more than a century and a half, such classifications are widely followed in back pain.[19]

We need to be aware that Virchow proposed that diseases came from abnormal activities inside the cells, not from outside pathogens. Since lower back pain is an epidemic in the modern world, Virchow needs to be given credit for the fact that he thought epidemics were social in origin, and he believed that the way to combat epidemics was political, not medical.

Soon enough came along the discovery of X-ray (1895) that could, for the first time, show the spine of a human being, without being cut open. Every coincidental finding on X-ray of the spine was sooner or later said to be the culprit for back pain. These findings brought along new diagnosis and justified the treatment prescribed by orthopaedics. This led to chronic back pain management being taken from a multidimensional (which wasn't always very helpful in getting rid of the pain) approach to a unidirectional physical approach. This at times worked fine, but aggravated the problem on the larger scale.

The two world wars resulted in phenomenal amount of casualties where the focus of attention shifted to accidents and trauma. Here, it was a lot easier to understand cause and effect, but this was somehow applied to everything in medicine and life.

Until then, back pain was just part of life. Bone-setting, or other recommendations for treating back pain were focused on getting the patient to carry on with life. Inadvertently, because of the circumstances that existed, orthopaedic practitioners put chronic back pain in a medical context; it suddenly became a disease and the sufferer became a patient. It ended up making them feel disabled.

In between the two world wars, the American Academy of Orthopaedic Surgery Commission on Back Pain reported in its survey that 'the general trend seems to be for longer and more complete bed rest'.[20]

Today, interventional treatments like injections and surgeries are offered very readily because of the advancement in these fields and also because of a very easy to understand and convincing cause-and-effect model. It's more probably because of instant gratification demanded by patients. In addition to that, recent research has shown that invasive treatment isn't better than conservative treatment.

Case: Saloni Khanna (name changed), sixty-five years old

A sixty-five-year-old homemaker complained of lower back pain for at least a week, before consulting a renowned orthopaedic surgeon in a popular corporate hospital. The senior doctor didn't even let her finish her story and told her that he knew all that was needed to be done. She was advised an MRI and in the same breath was told that there was a good chance that she would not be able to get back to her regular life if she didn't do as she was asked to. After looking at the MRI, the good doctor told her that her spine was hollow and was degenerating. She would need to get injections with imported medicines every month for the next twenty-four months. She was told that only he was certified to administer those injections in India. These injections would cost Rs 25,000 per month. Along with that, he would give her oral medicines for a month at the cost of Rs 15,000 per month. He also advised her to buy an imported lumbar belt that was only available with him. The doctor was very clear that if the patient didn't comply immediately, her condition would deteriorate very quickly and there was a good chance that she would be left paralysed. He wanted her to be completely bedridden for the next four to six months and be dependent on him.

Throughout the consultation, the patient or the patient's family didn't get a chance to speak. Here was a woman, who had managed her house for the last forty-five years; she had single-handedly looked after her husband, two sons and one daughter. She had been up and about for all these years, never really taking time to rest. She took the advice of bed rest as a death penalty.

What alerted the patient's family was the pushy behaviour of the doctor. They somehow stumbled upon my number. By the time she saw me, another four days had passed. The pain had already reduced by half. Upon examination, besides the apprehension of pain, everything else was normal. It took me half an hour to undo the damage done by my colleague. She simply had a muscle spasm because she had worked a bit too hard the day before the onset of pain. The pain had started because she was getting the house whitewashed. I advised her to go out twice a day for easy, slow walks for 10–15 minutes. Within a week, she was all fine. She came back and thanked me for having saved her 'life'. All I had done was offer her common-sense advice.

Unfortunately, along with good doctors, there are many such doctors around. But then such is the case in any field. Whether it be doctors or politicians, they are all part of the same society. We need to change ourselves to see the change happen in the society. Start with your own self. Move.

Why You Need This Book 17

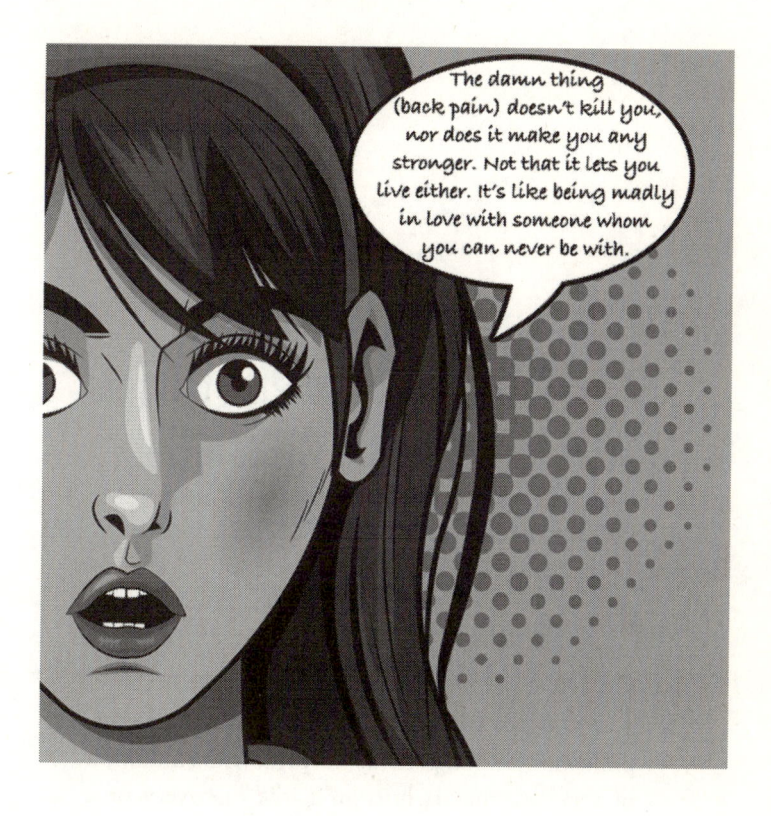

2

GETTING TO KNOW YOURSELF

Be an Alchemist

Alchemy: Merriam-Webster dictionary

noun
1. a medieval chemist science and speculative philosophy aiming to achieve the transmutation of the base metals into gold, the discovery of a universal cure for disease, and the discovery of a means of infidelity prolonging life
2. a power or process of transforming something common into something special

Genes Are Not Your Fate

Very often patients with back or knee pain report that either or both of their parents also had that pain. Almost always back and knee pains are not passed through generations.

Dean Ornish, a clinical nutrition professor at the University of California, San Francisco, and founder of the Preventive Medicine Research Institute, USA, stated in a TED Talk: 'Our genes are not our fate, and we make these changes—they're a predisposition, but if we make bigger changes than we might have made otherwise, we can actually change how our genes are expressed.'[1]

The above statement from Dr Ornish seems simultaneously optimistic and harsh, but is a simple fact that many are not aware of.

Respect Yourself, and the Rest Will Follow

You aren't simply a piece of furniture. You moved to be born and you were born to move. More importantly, you can feel and think. There is something that initiates your movement.

When any of us look at a skeleton, we feel scared. Of course, that skeleton can't do much on its own. There is no reason to be scared of the seemingly ever-smiling skeleton. Without ligaments, tendons and muscles, it can't move or be stable. It will simply topple over. The skeleton in a doctor's room has a rod inserted into the spine and wires that hold the various bones together.

The same applies to your back. It's simply not a skeleton. It is made to move and something initiates that movement. The thought that initiates movements should be in focus; only then movement of the body will happen.

Surprisingly, or not so surprisingly, most books on back pain start with explaining the spine, the bones (vertebrae) that form the spine, and the cushion (disc) between the vertebrae. The conventional view has been the assumption that pain in the back occurs from these structures, as discussed in the previous chapter. Once that thought is embedded in your mind, you will look only at the spine as the culprit for all your pains. When you start looking at yourself as a piece of furniture, you cannot blame the doctors for doing the same. You have ceased to exist as an intelligent human being who moves and has feelings too. You are just another patient with a pain in the back. The whole focus then is on your back and not on you.

That spine of yours is only a part of your body. It is true that the spine functions as the all-important chassis of your amazing body, but you are a lot more than just a physical body. You have to respect yourself before you expect the same from others.

You are an intelligent being, affected by your surroundings and environment. Even without wanting to, you absorb everything around you. You are a living being who moved, rather ran, to be born.

You Moved to Be Born

Let us go back in time—13.8 million years ago—when, leave alone life, time itself didn't exist. The earliest universe was highly energetic. It was replete with random movements that created this universe. The only constant in this universe is change; it's always moving. Does it not surprise you then, when you are told by the 'experts' not to move when you have back pain?

What is true of the universe is true of human beings too. A long time ago, before you were born, the sperm that formed part of you ran towards the egg. This led to the foetus being formed. Constant movement helped the foetus grow in size and also caused its neuro musculoskeletal growth, all of which plays a vital role in back pain. The foetus moves instinctively, to survive in its given environment.

What happened after that? Why did we all become such slobs and went against the basic rule of nature? We moved to be born. We need to keep moving to stay alive, else we will merely exist.

This puts everything else in our lives into perspective. It makes it clear that modern lifestyle and society are going against nature. Whether it is cosmology, physics or biology—movement created life. Somehow, in this modern world, we have forgotten to move. This is because the society around repeatedly tells us that it is 'normal' to not move, to be static slobs or pieces of furniture. This concept sticks with us and we start taking our bodies for granted.

Why Do We Need a Brain?

We need to first ask a fundamental question: Why do we need a brain? What is the reason that the brain exists in all of us? Knowing this will make you curious about how we go about catering to our pain. As I've said before, we aren't simply pieces of furniture, but we have been treated like that for long enough.

So, what's your guess? Why do we have a brain? Just pause and think about it. Maybe even discuss it with others in the room, or your Facebook friends. It's probably a good idea to tweet this question too. Just post it out there and come back to check the responses in a few hours. It'll be comforting for you to know that most folks are as clueless about this basic question as you are.

Daniel Wolpert, a Cambridge University neuroscientist, a self-confessed movement chauvinist, raised this basic but fundamental question during his TED Talk.[2] 'Why do we and other animals have a brain?' He and his team have spent their lives trying to answer this question. He suggests, 'We have a brain for one reason and one reason only, and that's to produce adaptable and complex movements. There is no other reason to have a brain. Think about it. Movement is the only way you have of affecting the world around you. But the clinching evidence is the humble sea squirt. This rudimentary animal has a nervous system and it swims around in the ocean in its juvenile life. And at some point of its life, it implants on a rock. And the first thing it does in implanting on that rock, which it never leaves, is to digest its own brain and nervous system for food. So once you don't need to move, you don't need the luxury of that brain. And this animal is often taken as an analogy to what happens at universities when professors get tenure, but that's a different subject.'

This openly challenges the conventional wisdom propagated by healthcare industry for over two-and-a-half centuries now, which discourages people to move.

Summation of Charles Darwin's theory of evolution is that it is not the strong of the species that survive, nor the most intelligent, but the one most responsive to change. Since the environment around us is always changing, we need to keep changing and moving to stay alive.

Now with this revelation, it'll make a lot more sense to stay mobile and moving, and disregard the wrong advice being given to you. To do justice to your body, you owe it to yourself to understand it better. It is of no interest to any other party to educate you. It is a waste of time for them.

What's in it for the healthcare industry to educate you to get you better and reduce their revenue? So, the onus is on you. It's your body. Know it better.

Role of the Mind in Dealing with Pain

'We will have pain when our brains "weigh the world" and "decide" that there is more danger to the body than safety.

We will not have pain when our brains "weigh the world" and "decide" that there is more safety related to the body than danger.'[3]

Harsheath, my fifteen-year-old son, reminded me of something on the above thought process. He narrated his experience at a science museum in Copenhagen about pain sensation and power of the brain. In a chamber, he was asked to touch a wall that was ice cold. He felt so cold touching it that it caused pain. Then he was asked to close his eyes and imagine himself on a beach on a sunny summer day where the temperature was perfect for swimming. Now he was asked to touch another wall. He didn't feel the wall to be as cold as the one before. He was then told that the temperature of both the walls was exactly the same. This time, he touched both the walls together and he felt both of them to be equally cold.

In simple terms, pain too can be a matter of perception. Your mind plays an important role in experiencing pain. Since it is you who perceives and experiences pain, it is logical to say that you can rid yourself of pain too. Either way, society and environment contribute immensely to the pain we experience.

The Body

Every time you think of back pain, you think about the bones in your back. Has it ever struck you that to move those bones and to stabilize joints, you need muscles, tendons and ligaments? Even my doctor colleagues, physiotherapists and other medical professionals, who treat back pain, do not seem to make an effort to convey this fundamental bit of information to their patient.

The skeleton, as scary as it might appear to people, cannot stay upright without muscles, tendons and ligaments.

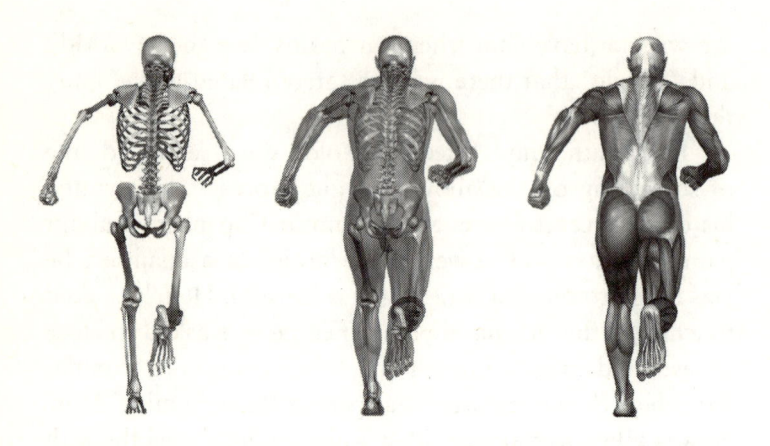

Our body would come tumbling down if it was not for the framework holding it up.

Spine works as a chassis of the body, the way it does in a car or a truck.

> A vehicle frame, also known as its chassis, is the main supporting structure of a motor vehicle to which all other components are attached, comparable to the skeleton of an organism. Until the 1930s, virtually every (motor) vehicle had a structural frame, separate from the car's body.—Wikipedia[4]

Case: Craig Longobardi, thirty-seven years old

Craig Longobardi, a thirty-seven-year-old flight mechanic, who performs helicopter search and rescue for the United States Coast Guard, shared his own story via email:

As someone having neck, back and vision issues, I've learnt a couple of things after having done some research. First was to learn how to explain what I'm feeling the way I do.

Someone else can't relate or understand the basics of what I've been going through.

As an endurance athlete, who has spent most of his life competing in marathons, numerous triathlons, 24-hour mountain bike races and so on, I understand pain. I also understand the difference between irritation and injury.

I found myself lacking the medical knowledge on how to fully describe what the issues were.

A couple of years ago, in the spring of 2014, I found myself in a particular dilemma.

I injured my neck and back while doing a daily chore. I felt a small pop in my neck. I didn't think anything of it at the time as it wasn't painful at all. Later that evening I started developing a headache. The next morning, I woke up with numbness in my right hand—this along with muscle spasms in my neck and back.

I took some basic over-the-counter drugs (Ibuprofen) and slept it off. The pain went away. A week later I saw a doctor. He sent me to a physical therapist. The symptoms would come and go if I did any activity. But I lacked the correct descriptions of what I felt. So I reverted to what I knew best and was common knowledge for most. I started describing my system as similar to an ordinary car. The frame being the skeleton; chassis being the spine; the engine being the heart; suspension being the discs between vertebrae bones; electrical wirings being the nerves, fuel being the oxygen, the car body being the skin, etc.

By working with the therapists and local doctors, I was able to understand what was wrong with my body. I also noticed that people were able to understand my problem better. The doctors told me that I had screwed up my chassis and the suspension which was causing short circuits in my electrical system. In medical jargon, I had bulging discs from the fourth cervical (C4) vertebrae through to seventh cervical vertebrae (C7), which were further indenting on my spinal cord.

Based on my experiences coupled with my background of being a mechanical engineer, I suggest that it's all right to screw up your car, but not your body, because you only have one body. A car can be repaired or its parts can be replaced. Worst-case scenario, you can just get a new car. Just that, we don't have that luxury with our bodies.

∼

Whether it is a car or a human body, you can't think about the back (spine) without thinking about the rest of the body, and you can't think of the body without thinking about the back (spine).

Between the muscles and skin is a connective layer called fascia. Think of this layer as an underwear for the whole body. Now, imagine when your underwear is even slightly off alignment. You feel uncomfortable throughout the whole day and are compelled to adjust it. If this underwear covers your entire body, it can go off alignment easily, leading to uncomfortable sensations throughout the day.

I bring this to your notice to make you aware that the back is more than just bones (vertebrae) in the spine and the discs in between, which are described below. You will be told repeatedly that discs are the main reason for your back pain. At times, it is the degenerating bones and discs that cause pain. That is not true. Most back pains are simply *dis-eases*. As soon as we remove the '*dis*', you will '*ease*' up.

Structures of the Spine

Contrary to popular belief, the spine is not an immobile straight rod. But shockingly, that's how it is treated even

Getting to Know Yourself

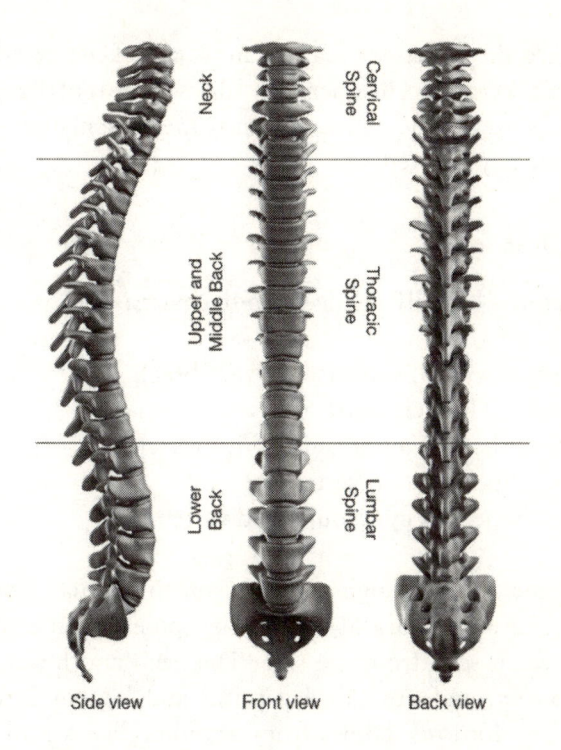

Figure: Side view (Neck, Upper and Middle Back, Lower Back); Front view (Cervical Spine, Thoracic Spine, Lumbar Spine); Back view.

by ones whom you trust with your health and back—the doctors and therapists. It's made to help you get from point A to B and beyond. Again, this cannot be done without the help of muscles, tendons and ligaments.

The spine's structure gives it function and its function determines its structure. What I mean is that if you have a good posture, it'll help you carry out all your activities optimally, whether it is walking, driving, working, playing with children and grandchildren, and so on. Staying active will, in turn, help your posture. For both of these to occur in sync, your spine needs to be in a good condition.

When we doctors talk to a patient about the human body, especially the spine, it is almost as if we are simply describing a piece of furniture, one that is doomed. We disregard the structures that are in place to keep everything dynamic. Vertebrae, ligaments and discs are part of the spine's passive system. The active system is the musculature—that is completely ignored.

Vertebrae

The spine is broadly divided into five parts:

1. Neck: Cervical spine (seven vertebrae)
2. Trunk: Thoracic spine (twelve vertebrae)
3. Lower back: Lumbar spine (five vertebrae)
4. Sacrum (five fused vertebrae)
5. Tail bone: Coccyx (four fused vertebrae)

The spine is not straight. Nothing in the human body is, nor in the whole natural world. The spine has an S-shaped curve when seen from the side. The neck and lower back are convex, and are called cervical and lumbar lordosis. The term 'lordosis' comes from 'standing like a lord', i.e., there is an exaggerated curve in the lower back and neck. The middle part of the spine is concave or kyphotic, to accommodate the vital organs, heart and lungs. Excessive concavity or convexity leads to problems.

The thirty-three vertebrae of different sections of the spine, mentioned above, are stacked on top of each other. The stacked vertebrae form a canal throughout the spine. We'll come to that later.

It is important for you to know more about the top three regions—cervical, thoracic and lumbar. They have their unique set of functions, which in case of imbalance can lead to unique dysfunctions (poor functioning) and injuries. This knowledge is important if you are trying to undo damage and lead a normal life.

Between any two vertebrae are discs, jelly-like shock absorbers. We will discuss that too later.

Neck: Cervical Spine

Very often, you will hear someone with neck pain say that 'they have a cervical'. You know what? All of us have cervical vertebrae, not one but seven. They are all in the neck region. The neck or cervical region is the most mobile of all the sections of the spine. The neck can bend to the side, rotate, bend forward as well as backward.

Upper and Middle Back: Thoracic Spine

The seven cervical vertebrae are stacked upon the twelve thoracic (or dorsal) vertebrae. Ribs are attached to the thoracic vertebrae, forming a ribcage. This ribcage is crucial to the protection of vital organs—heart and lungs. The shoulder blades are also attached to the ribcage through a number of muscles. Top 3–4 thoracic vertebrae also play a very important role in neck movements, specially forward bending. Upper thoracic region becomes very restricted, courtesy excessive usage of smartphones and computers.

Lower Back: Lumbar Spine

There are five lumbar vertebrae. The thoracic portion of the spine is stacked on these. Since this is a weight-bearing part of the spine, the lumbar vertebrae are bigger in size. Today's lifestyle leads to excessive back pain and the lumbar spine is the most affected in it. Repeated strain and load over long periods can injure this area. The movements facilitated by this portion of the spine are forward and backward bending.

Intervertebral Disc

In between any two consecutive vertebrae, there is an oval-shaped intervertebral disc. The discs play the role of shock absorbers to help absorb weight and pressure.

Think of the disc as a jam doughnut. The jam inside is contained by the outside layer of dough.

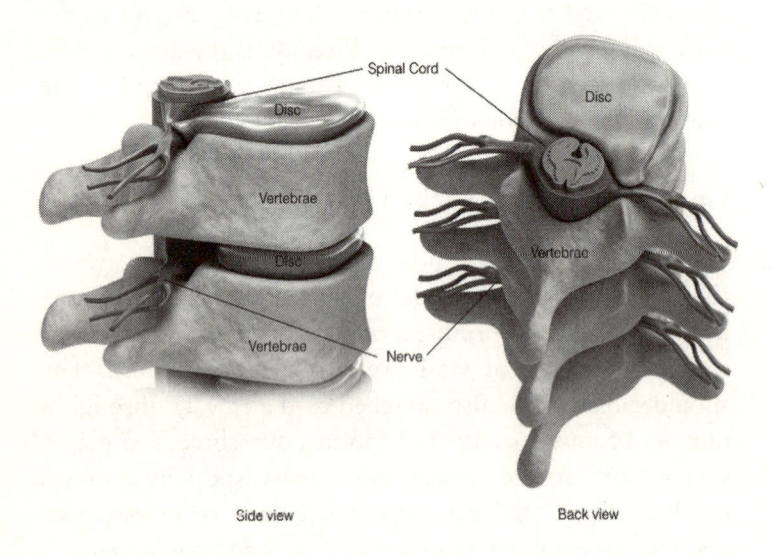

Side view

Back view

The jam-like inner part is called nucleus pulposus and the external dough part is called annulus fibrosus. Nucleus pulposus is a gel-like substance that consists of 88 per cent water, which gives the disc a pliable and flexible nature. Annulus fibrosus, on the other hand, is a fibrous cartilage layer, arranged in multiple onion-like layers around the inner part. Since the gel is towards the back of the disc, the annulus is weakest there and therefore the commonest site for tears and disc bulges. The strongest portion of the annulus is the front.

As we age, the discs become less pliable. The ligaments, muscles and tendons kick in to compensate for the loss of disc motility. This puts them under greater strain. Effectively, as you age, it becomes even more important to activate your muscles to prevent injuries.

Having said all that, it is important to note that as high as 66 to 75 per cent of adults above the age of thirty years who don't complain of any back pain, will have some disc bulge or the other, which is demonstrated on MRI.

Musculature

The muscular system constitutes 40 to 50 per cent of the body's total weight and is the single largest organ of the body. It is also the most underrated aspect of the human body. Muscles come into active use even before you are born, so that your growth can be normal. Muscles are needed to get out of the birth canal and then for your first breath and cry. Muscles help you move against gravity. Muscles are responsible for all your facial expressions.

On their own, the spine and skeleton cannot even hold themselves up. Muscles do that. Muscles help the body maintain its posture.

'The muscles, for the longest time, have been the "neglected children" of conventional medical care. No medical speciality actually focuses on treatment of the muscles.'[5] There is now a shift in this approach with the introduction of musculoskeletal medicine.

I really understood muscles for the first time when I was at the London College of Osteopathic Medicine. I started feeling them and listening to them. Experienced musculoskeletal medicine physicians and manual therapists (osteopaths, chiropractors, physiotherapists practising

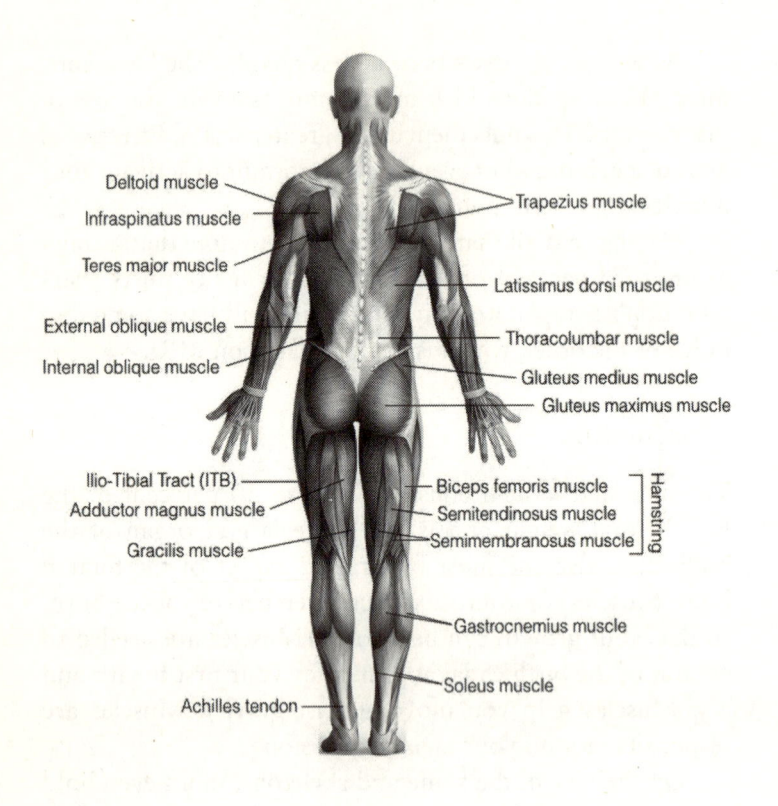

Figure: Posterior view of human musculature with labels: Deltoid muscle, Infraspinatus muscle, Teres major muscle, External oblique muscle, Internal oblique muscle, Ilio-Tibial Tract (ITB), Adductor magnus muscle, Gracilis muscle, Trapezius muscle, Latissimus dorsi muscle, Thoracolumbar muscle, Gluteus medius muscle, Gluteus maximus muscle, Biceps femoris muscle, Semitendinosus muscle, Semimembranosus muscle (Hamstring), Gastrocnemius muscle, Soleus muscle, Achilles tendon.

manual therapy, masseurs and so on) can touch and tell you, even before you say anything, where your pain is. There is nothing magical about it.

The doctor or therapist who does so repeatedly over the years can become good at this art. No high-tech investigation can pick up muscle spasms, but simple touch can. I got to know more about the function and role of musculature when I was heading the London centre of the medical department of Kieser Training, a Swiss-German strength-training chain of centres.

Muscles, ligaments and tendons not only hold up the spinal column, as well as the rest of the body, but they

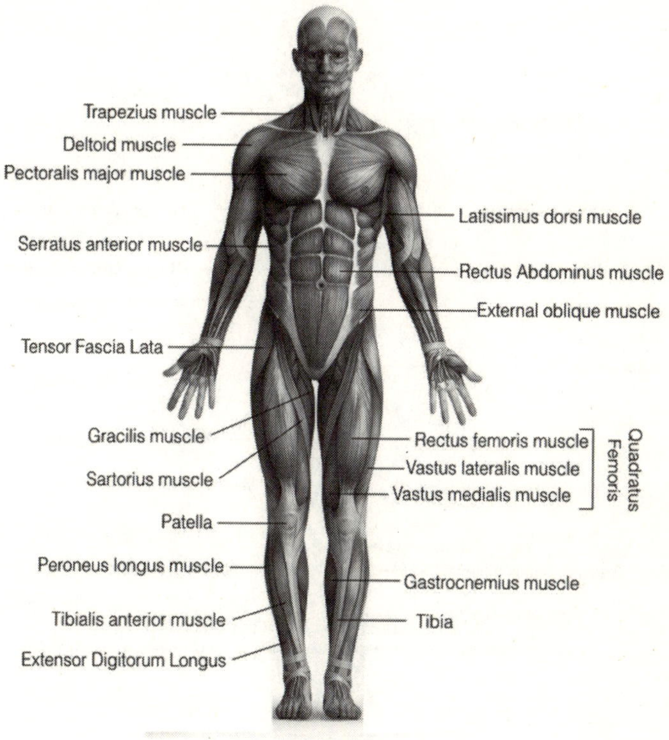
Trapezius muscle
Deltoid muscle
Pectoralis major muscle
Serratus anterior muscle
Tensor Fascia Lata
Gracilis muscle
Sartorius muscle
Patella
Peroneus longus muscle
Tibialis anterior muscle
Extensor Digitorum Longus
Latissimus dorsi muscle
Rectus Abdominus muscle
External oblique muscle
Rectus femoris muscle
Vastus lateralis muscle
Vastus medialis muscle
Quadratus Femoris
Gastrocnemius muscle
Tibia

also help move it. The skeleton alone can do nothing at all.

There is no one single magical muscle. All of them have to be in sync with each other to work. There is no need to remember their names. It is important to be aware where these muscles are and what they broadly do.

'The muscles are agents of movement and joint stability'.[6] This is also the case with those muscles that are around the spine. The smaller muscles that lie deeper and closer to the vertebral column help stabilize it. Both functions are important. The larger, longer muscles help directly or

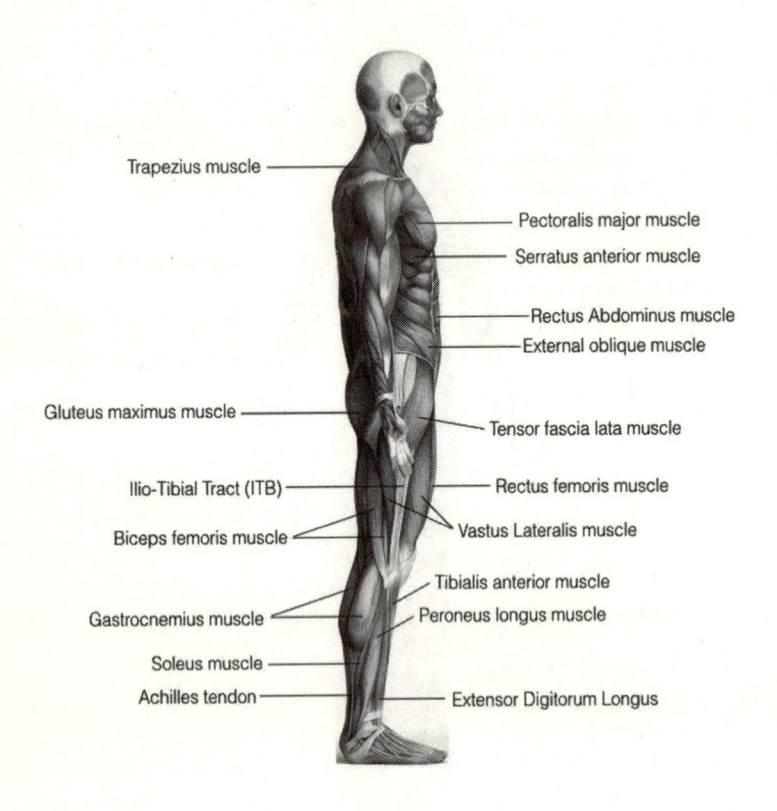

Figure labels:
- Trapezius muscle
- Pectoralis major muscle
- Serratus anterior muscle
- Rectus Abdominus muscle
- External oblique muscle
- Gluteus maximus muscle
- Tensor fascia lata muscle
- Ilio-Tibial Tract (ITB)
- Rectus femoris muscle
- Biceps femoris muscle
- Vastus Lateralis muscle
- Tibialis anterior muscle
- Gastrocnemius muscle
- Peroneus longus muscle
- Soleus muscle
- Achilles tendon
- Extensor Digitorum Longus

indirectly move the spine. Muscles around the spine, deep and superficial alike, form a corset around the spine.

All the muscles come together to play some role or the other in stabilizing the spine. Isn't it surprising that therapists and scientists pick a 'muscle of the season' every now and then. Every few months or years, there is a fascination with a particular muscle; that Eureka moment when a particular muscle is thought of as a miracle muscle responsible for stability. Once that is addressed, all kinds of pain will vanish. There is none. Think of the whole body when wanting to exercise the back, not just a new muscle every few months.

All the muscles of the body are important. When it comes to muscle movement, there is no need to complicate matters. Imagine A and B to be the two ends of a muscle. When the muscle contracts, A and B move towards each other over the shortest distance possible. So, when you do any exercise, you first need to know which muscle you are activating, as well as the action of that muscle. That is what you should focus on. All other body parts need to completely relax while you are doing the exercise.

Spinal Cord and Nerves

As mentioned above, all the vertebrae are stacked upon each other in such a way that they form a canal from top to bottom. Through this canal passes the sensitive, snake-like structure called the spinal cord, which is an extension of the brain. The spinal cord further gives out spinal nerves at each vertebral level, which exit the canal at corresponding vertebral levels. These spinal nerves, from each level, supply different muscles (myotome) and skin areas (dermatome) of the body. If a particular nerve is irritated because of impingement, there can be pain down the affected nerve's course or weakness of the muscles.

The area of the skin supplied by a single spinal nerve is called a dermatome. Spinal nerves from the neck (cervical) region primarily supply the skin of the back of the head, neck and arms. Spinal nerves of the upper back (thoracic) region supply the upper back and the torso. Spinal nerves of the lower back (lumbar) region supply the front of the legs and the soles of the feet, whereas spinal nerves from the sacral region supply the back of the legs.

Each muscle in the body is supplied by one or more levels or segments of the spinal cord and by their corresponding spinal nerves. A group of muscles innervated by the motor fibres of a single nerve root is known as a myotome.

A radiating pain, which is pain along the course of a particular nerve, can be caused if the spinal nerves are injured or trapped anywhere along their course. The most popular kind of radiating pain is 'sciatica', which is pain that travels down the length of a leg. It can also cause a pins-and-needle or numbness sensation along the course of the spinal nerve. The sensation to touch could also be different in a particular area. Radiating pain can also lead to muscle weakness corresponding to the spinal nerve(s) involved.

You need to remember that the spinal cord and nerves are like politicians the world over, slippery and slimy. Spinal cord occupies only one third of the diameter of the spinal canal. The spinal cord might get impinged by the disc bulge and cause pain, but soon enough the spinal cord frees itself by finding open space.

Movements of the Spine

Spine Movements

None of the vertebrae are flat bones. They are like a jigsaw puzzle that fit perfectly into each other. The back of each vertebra has two pairs of bony processes lined with cartilage, one pair facing upwards, the other downwards. These are called 'facet joints'. They are plate-like structures that link the vertebrae above and below. The direction of facet joints determines the movements available at each vertebrae level.

Each facet joint is enclosed in a capsule which contains synovial fluid, this in turn provides lubrication and nutrition to the joint cartilage. Repeated incorrect or excessive movement at each facet joint can cause the capsule to become overstretched, leading to more movement at that joint.

Neck/Cervical Spine

The skull is placed upon the cervical spine. The cervical spine (neck) is the most mobile part of the spine; it can rotate and bend on the sides, forward and backward. It is in turn placed upon the thoracic spine, which is the least mobile part of the spine. This fact makes the junction between the two highly prone to injuries.

Upper and Middle Back/Thoracic Spine

Protection offered to vital organs by the ribcage limits the movements of the thoracic portion of the spine. The bones at this level are designed in such a way that rotation movements happen here. When you sit down and rotate left or right, most of that movement should happen at the thoracic level. Thoracic spine plays a very crucial role in sports like golf, tennis, fast bowlers in cricket, any throws, etc. Poor posture leads to stiff upper and middle back, and the rotational movement that should have happened at thoracic spine takes place at lumbar spine. This is a recipe for disaster.

Lower Back/Lumbar Spine

This is the most important part of the spine pertaining to back pain. The direction of facet joints in this part only allows forward and backward bending. Poor posture can lead to the stiffening of the thoracic spine (middle back). Sportsmen like golfers, fast bowlers in cricket, tennis players, etc., put the spine through immense pressure while rotating. The lumbar spine (lower back) tries to compensate for the lack of rotation in the thoracic spine (middle back) by trying to do the rotations, even though that is not its function. Over time, this can lead to a stress fracture in the lower back. Stress fracture is common amongst younger athletes who have a poor posture coupled with muscle imbalance. If attention is not paid, a complete fracture can also occur in the lower back.

Spring-like Character

Intervertebral discs, along with the S-shaped curve, function like shock absorbers when pressure is put on the spine while doing activities like walking, running or jumping. Both of them together give the spine its springiness.

The spine forms an exaggerated 'S' when pressure is put on it and then bounces back to its normal shape. Most of us, as we age, abuse our bodies, which leads to a distortion of our natural curves. The natural springiness of the spine is also compromised. Each impact on the spine leads to the body having a compensatory protective response.

Muscles go into spasms as an immediate response; but if it recurs over time, it causes pain. The protective, compromised posture might also become a habit of the muscle, leading to chronic pain. The problem is that most doctors only treat pain symptomatically, without addressing the underlying cause. After triggering muscles the wrong way, the main problem might have disappeared; but only after leaving behind gross muscle imbalance and poor posture. Now, it becomes a chronic condition. One problem feeds off the other.

This book will try to address the underlying causes of poor posture and muscle imbalances, as 80–90 per cent of pain can be addressed by simply doing that. And it's a lot simpler than you would have imagined.

Functions of the Spine: All Systems Work in Sync

The spine has to be both flexible and stable. It is participating in a balancing act between different forces all the time. As suggested earlier, similar to the chassis of an automobile, flexibility (mobility) and stability together provide protection to the spinal cord and nerves.

It is the constant harmony between stability and mobility that makes the spine special.

For the entire body to perform optimally, both characteristics of the spine are needed together—in the right balance and the right amount. Lack of either will not only lead to injury but will also prevent you from functioning optimally, whether it is sitting in front of the television or computer or playing football.

The legs and arms are like wheels that will only work optimally if the chassis, or the spine in this case, is perfectly aligned. Isn't it surprising that in most exercise programmes, whether it is for amateurs or elite professional sportspersons, the spine almost never gets the attention it deserves? Time and again, I have come across so-called gym instructors and bodybuilders who have spines weaker than mine.

The spine needs to be stable when we run but, at the same time, it needs to be immensely mobile to make the experience smooth. Golf, among all sports, is the best example of perfect synchronization of mobility and stability to help the body perform better.

Injury usually starts much earlier, with *dys-function*; this effectively refers to the body not functioning at an optimal level. There is no *disease* yet, but there is *dis-ease*. *Dis-ease* and *dys-function* feed off each other, pulling the body into a vicious circle. Conventional doctors are unable to deal with this situation as they are only trained to treat disease, sickness and injury. Also, the imbalance between mobility and stability could lead to the reversal of what the function of the spine is. So instead of protecting the delicate spinal cord and nerve roots, it could start irritating and damaging them. Soon enough, there will be an injury too.

Neuro Musculoskeletal System

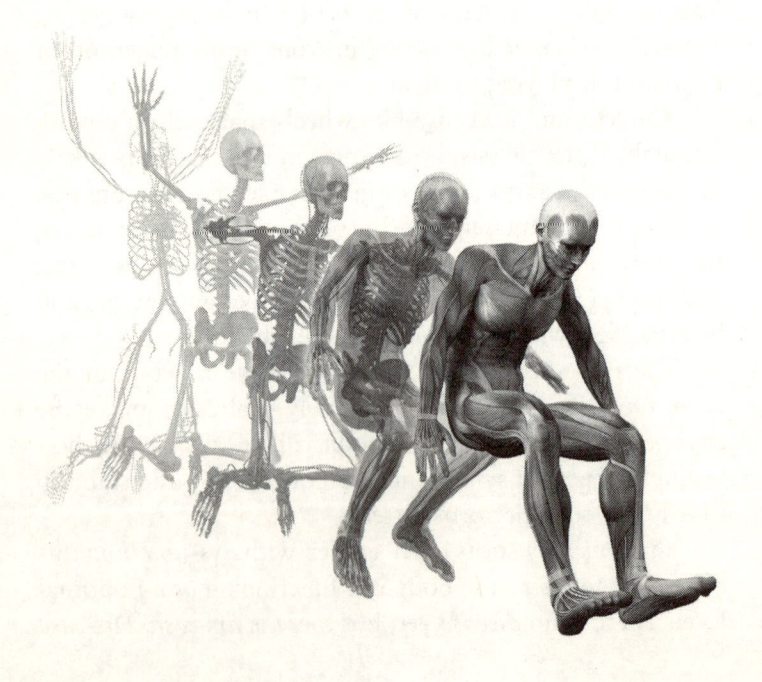

The vertebral column alone, without the support of muscles, ligaments and tendons, with the vertebrae stacked on top of each other, can buckle under less than 9 kg of weight. However, on a regular basis, the vertebral column bears loads that are twenty times greater than this. These are encountered while doing daily activities like sitting, standing, lifting a weight, or even lying down.

Dr Manohar Panjabi,[7] way back in 1992, said, 'This large load-carrying capacity is achieved by the participation of well-coordinated muscles surrounding the spinal column.' We now know it is the neuro musculoskeletal system as a whole that needs to work properly, to enable us to optimally use the body.

I like to think of our body as the most sophisticated machine ever created. For the sake of comprehending better, with all due respect to the rest of the world, let us call it a state-of-the-art Swiss–German machine. The skeleton is like the mainframe of that machine. The musculature is similar to various levers present in that machine that help in its movement.

As beautiful as it might look, it can do nothing without electricity. The nervous system is like the electric supply. Now if someone cuts off the electric supply, the machine can't move even a single millimetre or degree. In case of a short circuit, the machine might stop working altogether.

All movements and pain are controlled by the brain. It is the nerves that carry messages from the brain to the spinal cord, and further to various parts of the body.

The skeleton plays an important role in protecting the delicate nervous system. The brain is protected within the skull, whereas the spinal cord is protected within a canal formed by the vertebrae and an encapsulating sheath called the dura mater.

To add to that, Craig Liebenson[8] has rightly observed:

> Surprisingly, the motor control system functions well under load. Muscles stabilize joints by stiffening like

rigging on a ship. But, when load is at minimum, such as when the body is relaxed or a task is trivial, the motor control system is often caught off guard; and injuries are precipitated.

Here, the muscles are not doing much, but similar problems occur if muscles, ligaments and tendons have been under excessive load for long durations. What is desirable is 'optimal load'.

Usually, doctors and patients try to put a finger on that one incident that caused the injury. Lower back pain is not the result of any one injury. Even if it seems like it, that injury is most probably the proverbial last straw on the camel's back. The conditions that enabled the injury have probably been building up for years.

Professor Stuart McGill,[9] an authority in spine biomechanics, points out that 'it usually is a result of excessive loading which gradually, but progressively, reduces the tissue failure tolerance'. In simple terms, what it means is that excessive load over long durations on the spine lowers the tolerance level at which tissues get injured.

Posture

> Even on the highest throne in the world, we are still sitting on our ass.
>
> —Michel de Montaigne

Since you now know about the neuro musculoskeletal system a lot more than most doctors treating your aches and pains, let's raise the bar a little. Just having the right tools won't help if you don't know what to do with them.

Posture[10] is a complex mixture of individual structure, habits of mind and body, movement patterns, breathing and complex activities of the nervous system.

Start with becoming aware of what a good posture is, so that everything else can fall into place. Postural improvement starts with awareness of your body. Be aware that posture is a dynamic balance of your whole body, especially head, neck and back. 'Back' is really a misnomer as there is no marked demarcation between the behind and front, both structurally and functionally. Your skull sits on your neck, which sits on your thorax, which is on the lumbar region, which in turn is on the pelvis and sacral regions. The ribcage is attached to the thorax, which literally forms a cage for sensitive organs—heart and lungs.

All three (head, neck, back) need to be in perfect harmony with each other at all times, day or night. It should be irrespective of what you are doing—lying down, sitting, standing, walking, running, swimming, playing a sport and so on.

You have to learn how to sit and stand straight by 'releasing' the tension and letting go, rather than 'imposing' a forced posture. That'll help in maintaining the new posture. It needs to be effortless. It's an ongoing process, a fine balance. It's almost like trying to balance a snooker, pool or billiard cue on one finger. The harder you try, the more difficult it is. The more relaxed you are, the easier it is. You need to be mindful though.

It'll be tough initially, but soon it'll become second nature.

In their eagerness to fix the problem, some doctors and therapists might ask you to force yourself to have all three (head, neck and back) in one straight line. Instead of relieving pain, this might make you even more uncomfortable. Soon, it'll cause you even more pain.

We need to understand that when we talk about good posture, it's not simply about the position of bones and joints in relation to each other. Muscles, ligaments, tendons and fascia keep our bones and joints in the position that they are in. For the longest time, we've been told to sit with our backs ramrod straight. We force ourselves to sit or stand in a position that is actually more uncomfortable, as the basic foundation hasn't been corrected. In any case, we will not be able to hold that position for very long.

The muscles, ligaments, tendons and fascia need to be well balanced for you to have a good posture. A sedentary lifestyle and working long hours at a desk can affect your posture. It'll change your posture for worse, even if you had a good posture before you joined your well-paying but sedentary job. Ideally, you need to find a new job, but this is not a perfect world. We need to figure out realistic solutions in the given settings, and keep you employed as well.

Breathing

As long as you live, you'll breathe and you'll have some sort of a posture, whether good or bad. Like breathing, posture is a dynamic process. Good posture leads to optimum breathing, and vice versa.

The lungs are the organs that are used for breathing. Think of the lungs as balloons with a shell around it. Ribcage is the shell around the lungs.

Lungs sits on a muscle called 'diaphragm'. The diaphragm is an important muscle for breathing, but for a long time it has been treated as the only muscle that is needed or works in breathing. There are a lot of other muscles that are either directly or indirectly involved in breathing.

When you breathe in, the lungs try to expand in all directions, similar to a balloon. For the balloon to expand optimally, the surrounding shell also needs to expand sideways, in front and back. To do this, the ribs should, simultaneously, flare outwards and lift slightly.

Ribs have a bucket-handle-like action where the bucket handle in front is attached to the breastbone (sternum) and at the back to the thoracic spine.

If you maintain a poor posture, the lungs will not have enough space to expand. For the same reason, poor breathing will directly lead to a poor posture. This becomes a vicious cycle, leading to a bad habit for life. This will affect every physical activity you'll do by limiting your breathing and movement capacity.

It's estimated that the earliest evidence of oxygen-breathing organisms dates back to nearly 2.5 billion years. Without oxygen none of us would exist, definitely not in the current form. We are too busy thinking about the possibility of life existing elsewhere in the universe, but we are ignoring the one life that we are sure about, the one that we have been gifted. We first need to appreciate it and do justice to it, before thinking about life elsewhere.

I would like to compare each breath to a bus and lungs to bus stops. If you take quick, shallow breaths, it's equivalent to the bus not stopping for long enough for its passengers to board (inhale oxygen) or alight (exhale carbon dioxide). By taking shallow breaths, you are only using the upper part of your lungs. And in that portion of the lung, there's a minimal amount of oxygen–carbon dioxide exchange. But when you take deep, controlled breaths, it's equivalent to the bus spending the optimum amount of time at the 'stop' for the necessary exchange of oxygen and carbon dioxide.

To add to this, imagine a barrier around the bus stop that makes it difficult for the carbon dioxide to get off, and for the oxygen to get in. That's exactly what is going on within most of us. We hold our torso too tight and don't let our ribs expand with each breath. Our shoulders are held up or bent forward. Breathing is shallow because it is quick and vice versa. This contributes to back pain.

When the head and torso are forced in an upright position by tight and tense muscles or a bad posture, they end up constricting the movement of the ribs. To begin with, the capacity of your lungs to expand is limited. Poor posture leads to poor body habits and vice versa. In most adults, when asked to take deep breaths, there is minimal movement of the ribs.

Muscles of the neck, torso and back are directly involved with what the ribcage can or cannot do. They determine how freely the diaphragm moves. While breathing in, the diaphragm moves down and the ribcage expands by going up and out. If your body is being pulled down and all surrounding muscles in the neck, torso and back are tense, they won't let the lungs expand.

Sitting for long periods at a stretch makes your hamstrings and psoas muscles to remain in a shortened position. Soon, this becomes the comfortable length for both the muscles. Once shortened muscle length becomes second nature to the body, it is difficult to counter it. The shortened muscles force the pelvis to move down, putting immense pressure on the lower back muscles. Over time, this puts you in a posture that seems like the most comfortable one, which is either a C-shaped spine or an exaggerated S-shaped spine while lying down, sitting and standing. If your starting posture is wrong, when you start moving, the same will persist.

Your body will make compensatory changes in an effort to get to the right posture, but each effort will only make the posture worse, putting undue pressure on the body. It might not hurt right away, but soon you'll start getting all kinds of pains. When you meet someone like me, you'll ask the question that most people with pain ask, 'How did this happen to me?'

Breathing out is equivalent to the shell shrinking—the diaphragm rises and the ribcage comes together. This helps in exhaling as well. If you don't exhale out, your lung capacity will be reduced. Even though not enough is spoken about it, this is an equally important part of breathing.

Had you allowed your body to breathe properly by having a good posture, it would not have deteriorated so much, so soon. It's you alone who has the power to fix this problem. It's definitely not too late; it never is.

Let's do a little experiment. Sit down in your most comfortable posture, not bothering if it is the right one. You've become an expert at it as you've been doing it for as long as you can remember. Go ahead, slouch, bring your head forward, your shoulders in front, lean back against the backrest, slide down the chair. If you fancy having your feet on the table or putting one atop another, don't think twice. Just do it, it's your body, go ahead and abuse it.

Now take long, deep breaths in. And then out. Repeat a few times, till you think you are little less conscious about it. You'll see that even if you are not aerodynamic and well rounded, it'll still be your tummy that will go up and down with each long breath. Now look what your chest does when you take those deep breaths. Surprisingly, it doesn't move much. Among most people, it'll be very still.

Every time you breathe out, along with your tummy going up, your head, neck and thorax collapse down into your tummy. It doesn't help that there is poor tone of spine musculature and belly.

If we were to record just your chest movement while you were busy taking deep breaths in and out, and show it to you later, I'm pretty sure you'll not be able to make out if you were dead or alive. Now stop playing dead, and start living by doing justice to that one body that you have been given. Learn to breathe properly, for starters.

If your posture and body aren't good, your breathing can't be good either. You need to improve your posture and body to have any chance of improving your breathing.

Mouth vs Nose for Breathing

There is no comfortable shortcut to success. If one appears, check again because you might be on the wrong track. The same applies to breathing from the mouth while you are not doing any strenuous activity like running or playing a sport. A lot more air might go in when you breathe from the mouth, but you end up stiffening your ribs. Since your lungs now have limited space to expand in the stiff ribcage, you can't take long breaths. You try to compensate for it by increasing the frequency of breathing, but that makes your breaths shallow.

When you breathe in through your nose, it takes longer and hence is harder than breathing through your mouth. That's the reason why many people prefer breathing from their mouths.

Case: Vikas Rana (name changed), forty-two years old

A top-notch lawyer came with severe lower back pain that he had for four days, with stiffness for the last three months. He needed treatment because his back pain had suddenly increased and he was to fly to Europe in less than a week.

On examination, it was discovered that there was a disc bulge irritating a spinal nerve. I needed to find a solution that would rid him of pain immediately and help him stay pain-free even after coming back. I noticed that while breathing, he would not use his torso at all. His ribs were not expanding on being asked to take deep breaths. He would easily get stressed and his posture showed a lot of tension in his neck, shoulders and lower back. His neck was jutting forward, with raised and rounded shoulders, sunken breastbone and a slumped posture.

I only asked him to focus a little more on his breathing, and his back pain was already better the next morning. He was then asked to concentrate a little more on letting go and not stiffening up to sit straight.

Suddenly, there was a marked drop in the severity of his back pain. During the long flight to Europe he practised relaxed and easy breathing. He had no difficulty walking around in Europe only because he was made to understand his situation and how he could address it. Normally, someone like him would have been advised to cancel the trip and most probably undergo surgery.

Psychology in Posture and Movement

Emotional and psychological conditions are expressed physically. You would have often heard of the term 'body language'. It can change when you are in a particular frame of mind, but over a period of time it can become a habit.

If you are holding tension in your neck, shoulder and upper back, you need to deal with it before exercising. Else, exercise will only make the condition worse.

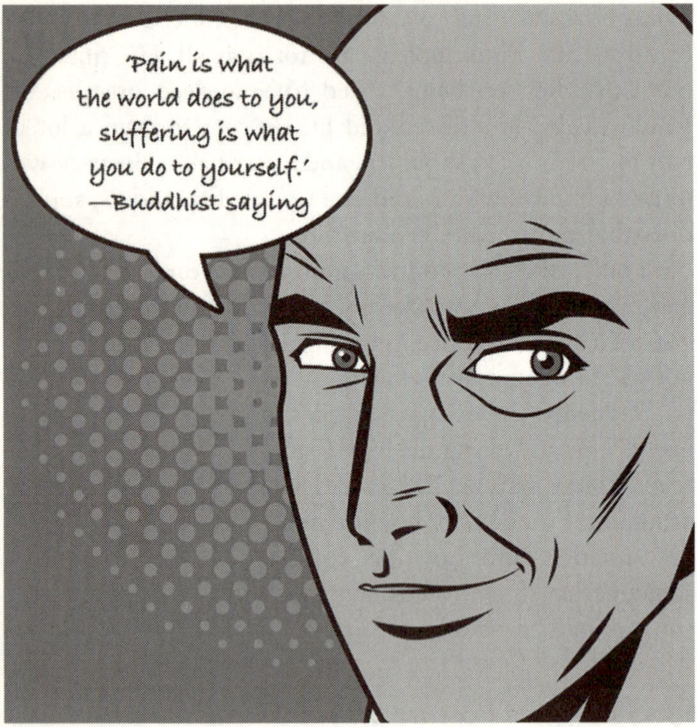
'Pain is what
the world does to you,
suffering is what
you do to yourself.'
—Buddhist saying

3

WHAT YOU SHOULD DO WHEN YOU HAVE BACK PAIN

Most doctors treat you like a piece of furniture.
Good ones understand that you were made to move.
Amazing ones appreciate that you can think and feel too.
This, I am a firm believer of.

Doctors and Therapists

An overwhelming majority of people suffering from back pain do not have a serious medical condition, or one that needs them to stop all movement.

Today, top doctors and international back pain guidelines are of the consensus that bed rest is actually detrimental. Almost always, pain is out of proportion to how serious the condition is, i.e., a lot more than how serious the disease is. Also, people either become too apprehensive or treat it too casually. You need to be better informed, but not via the Internet. Doctor Google can confuse matters even more as there is no way of knowing the credibility of the person who has written the information.

My earnest request to anyone suffering from pain, whether recent or chronic, is to calm down. Your pain is almost always greater than the magnitude of the actual damage. The more you stress about it, trust me, the worse your pain will become.

Take long breaths, don't panic and don't take a cafeteria approach, which means don't keep consulting all kinds of doctors till you find the one who suggests what you want to hear. You'll eventually find someone who'll do or advise what you want. Don't look for the most popular names. What you are looking for is good advice, which is not biased by your thoughts.

Treat All Humans as Equals and Be Treated as an Equal Too

Most doctors will tell you what you shouldn't do when suffering from back pain, but will not tell you what you should do to manage it. Unintentionally, they put you in a passive role, which you have actually chosen. You will only be treated as an equal if you start treating your doctors as equals. Mostly patients put them on an unnecessary pedestal. Respect doctors, but don't turn them into demigods. Remember, power corrupts. Else, be prepared to be treated like an inferior race by my colleagues. It's difficult for anyone to stay grounded once they have been placed on a pedestal. However, this does not mean you should not respect your doctors. Don't suspect them of trying to fleece you. They are human too and happen to belong to the same society as you. They are what the society is. The change has to start with you.

Case: M. Radhakrishnan (name changed), thirty-five years old

A thirty-five-year-old army officer consulted me for back pain. He came with an X-ray. His back pain had persisted for more than three to four months and he wasn't able to perform his regular duties and daily household chores. I requested an MRI, which I rarely do but then they are needed at times. There was a stress fracture in one of his lumbar vertebrae, leading to instability. I asked the patient to share the same MRI with his doctor at the army hospital. Unfortunately, the army doctor didn't like that a civilian doctor had ordered an MRI, when he hadn't asked for one. He chose to make it an ego clash, and ignored the findings of the MRI. He ordered the army officer back to his post sooner than I think was appropriate. He needed more rest.

Such ego clashes are common in the medical fraternity. Sadly, it's the patient who always loses in such cases.

Names, Do They Really Matter?

> Doctors are men who prescribe medicines of which they know little, to cure diseases of which they know less, in human beings of whom they know nothing.
>
> —Voltaire (1694–1778)

Richard P. Feynman, ranked as one of the ten greatest physicists of all times, said something no doctor should ever forget:

> You can know the name of a bird in all the languages of the world, but when you are finished, you'll know

absolutely nothing whatsoever about the bird. So let's look at the bird and see what it's doing—that's what counts. I learned very early the difference between knowing the name of something and knowing something.

Medicine is an amalgamation of art and science. However, contemporary medicine lacks the element of art. In our eagerness to become tech-savvy, we have forgotten the basics of medicine. It's almost as if science is trying to catch up with art. Sometimes to understand and appreciate our own subject better, we need to look elsewhere.

'I've learned that people will forget what you said, people will forget what you did, but people will never forget how you made them feel,' these are the amazing words of author Maya Angelou that all doctors should implement during their consultations and interactions with their patients.

Since we doctors are trained really well to pass exams, and are good at knowing all kinds of random names of diseases, it doesn't necessarily mean that we understand them well enough. Musculoskeletal medicine is a field that suffers from this malaise. We doctors happily put various kinds of tags on patients based on our limited knowledge. Soon enough, the patients show all the symptoms appropriate for that disease because they have been consulting Dr Google on a regular basis. With all good intentions, we end up creating more problems than we solve.

Choosing the Right Doctor/Therapist

This is a million dollar question.

Let me start by telling you how you could have approached this issue in a perfect world.

Ideally, family doctors or general physicians should be the first point of contact for any illness. They should be like the 'gatekeepers' of the healthcare industry. The same applies to pain. It's their job to figure out the future plan of action based on the severity of your pain. They might give you some medication, investigate or directly refer you to a specialist, based on their judgement. Almost always, they adopt a conservative approach, do not rush into investigations, and rarely ever prescribe injections and surgeries.

Unfortunately, the family doctor culture has disappeared and general physicians are rare to come by any longer. The situation has been created by both 'demand' and 'supply'. We all want to be seen by specialists. We end up going to them and then complain that they ask for investigations or do procedures that are not needed. We ignore the fact that they have been trained to focus on particular types of pains, which might be more complicated than the problem at hand. They also don't want to miss out on anything serious. Before complaining, remember that they didn't come to you. It was you who wanted to go to a specialist right in the beginning.

The dip in demand of general physicians has made doctors focus on specializing. Not many are now able to address the commonest cause of back pain, which doesn't need any investigations or procedures.

So, what should be your strategy in the current set-up where there aren't enough family doctors or general physicians?

When in pain, you need a doctor who will listen to you and understand your problem, more than a doctor with a speciality. You should pick a doctor you know will listen or one who has a reputation of doing exactly that. You would assume that all doctors would be like that. Yes, in an ideal world, they should be. The physical factors of pain trigger psychological factors and vice versa, which feed off each other. The doctor needs to be able to understand and appreciate this aspect of the disease too.

We all might have come across technically sound doctors who are impolite and not ready to listen. There are doctors who start writing a prescription in less than a minute of your having entered the consultation room. If you continue with your complaints, they give you a last warning. If you make the mistake of asking any more questions after that, you have to leave the consultation room. These individuals hold top positions in the medical fraternity and have worked in premier institutions for decades. Such characters don't give you much confidence. However, such doctors exist across specialities.

Then there are doctors who can scare the living daylights out of you. They'll make it sound as if it's the end of the world. As mentioned earlier, at almost all times pain is inevitable but suffering is optional. This is easier said than done. Your doctor or therapist needs to help you tackle pain better, so there is less suffering.

You need to look for a doctor who has a reputation of hearing you out and is not in a rush. When you have pain, you have a lot to share. Sometimes, that's all you really need to do. Appropriate medical advice is then a bonus.

Listening Skills

Doctors in the US interrupt their patients within 12 seconds, in 28 seconds in Slovenia and Croatia, and in 47 seconds in the UK. When a patient with long-standing pain presents it to a doctor, he expects to be listened to, but sadly almost all doctors are in a rush.

Doctors will only be able to 'listen' if they are 'silent'. That's a bit difficult for us doctors because we have too little time and too much to share. Listening will simply not happen if we keep interrupting patients. Almost all of my colleagues are ready with advice even before you are done.

No amount of forms being filled at hospitals or clinics can replace what the patient has to say to a doctor. If the patient feels that the doctor understands him, half of the issues are taken care of. It is important to talk. If a doctor can't listen to you, he definitely needs to be in the back office. Listening to the patient must be followed up with asking relevant questions to get a better idea of what is going on.

Case: Seema Arora (name changed), fifty-eight years old

A shy fifty-eight-year-old homemaker from Delhi had been complaining of lower back pain since two decades. She had seen numerous doctors and had got several investigations done.

She had episodes of severe back pain which lasted 10–15 days. The pain was not always excruciating. Even on examination, there was nothing that clearly explained her symptoms. I had to talk to her again to ask details of her family and lifestyle. She had spent the last three decades looking after everyone at home. Even though she is very active throughout the day, she can't find time to go for walks.

Soon enough she was not so much complaining about her back pain but about her mother-in-law who constantly nagged her. However, her relationship with her twenty-seven-year-old daughter was very good and she enjoyed her company.

I advised her to take a week-long holiday with her daughter. This was her first vacation since she had been married. They both visited Bengaluru and Arora didn't complain of pain after she got back. She understood the importance of 'me time' and for once she is focusing a bit on herself too. Now she goes for regular walks and has started yoga as well.

Human Touch

Human touch, whether it is for clinical examination or treatment, is a lost art in modern 'conventional' medicine. Dr Abraham Verghese, professor of the theory and practice of medicine at Stanford University, US, and a writer, during his TED talk said that we live in a strange new world where patients are merely data points, and called for a return to the traditional one-to-one physical examination. He says, 'I still find the best way to understand a (hospitalized) patient is not by staring at the computer screen but by going to see the patient; it's only at the bedside that I can figure out what is important.'

He goes on to remind us that 'prior to that time (discovery of auscultation and percussion in clinical examination) no matter what ailed you, you went to see the barber surgeon who wound up cupping you, bleeding you, purging you. And, oh yes, if you wanted, he would give you a haircut—short on the sides, long in the back—and pull your tooth while he was at it. He made no attempt at diagnosis.'

Have we doctors gone back to those practices? Leave alone surgeons, even physicians are no less guilty of the same.

These days, even physiotherapists (physical therapists) are not trained how to touch, when that should be fundamental for them. A majority of them have become electrotherapists, when they should have been physical therapists. Their work should at least involve manual work (examining and treating with hands) and exercise (as a modality to treat patients).

It almost seems plausible or maybe wishful thinking by Dr Verghese, that the most important innovation in medicine to come in the next ten years would be 'the power of the human hand'. Touché!

No high-tech investigation can yet examine the body's functioning like a good, old-fashioned physical examination. It starts from the best tool that all doctors need to work on—touch. My examination starts from the waiting area. Besides observing the patient's posture while sitting and gait while walking, I also shake the patient's hand. That one act does a lot of good. It gives the patient confidence in me and builds a rapport.

Only once did a patient not shake my hand. It was a lady in a burka in London. Since then, I am a bit more sensitive to cultural differences. After listening to the patient's story, only if I have some questions do I ask them at that point.

I also look at the patient's shoes. We all spend more than half our lives in them. Shoes almost always talk back to me, and they never lie. They tell me what the patient's body has been putting them through. If the shoes aren't comfortable, chuck them right now. They are not meant for you.

Then I get my patients to stand and inspect their back, side and front. Only when I have had a good look, do I start examining the back. During my examination of the back, I look at a range of movements of the spine and do other physical tests while the patient is standing, sitting, lying on the back, on the side and finally face down on his or her abdomen.

Now, this ritual takes around 10 minutes, but it often tells me more than most high-tech investigations. I don't have X-ray vision, but X-rays know nothing about the things that move the skeletal system, muscles, tendons, ligaments, fascia and so on. I am interested in looking at the whole patient, and not only the painful back. Broadly, I like to assess the posture (gait while walking, standing, sitting and lying down), breathing, body movements, among others.

Basically, what I have looked at is what is functioning well in the body. Once I know your strengths, it is easier for me to address your weaknesses. The basic premise is that the body always makes an effort to be normal and function optimally; it just needs to be shown the right direction as to how to get there.

After assessing the patient at the macro level, I look at the patient at a micro level to confirm or rethink my original observations. I assess muscle imbalances, muscle strength and weakness, muscle activation, muscle tightness, a range of motion of joints, their stability or instability, and so on.

The buzz word nowadays is functional examination or functional training, but we also need to be aware of the strongest and weakest links in the chain to have a better treatment plan.

After I am done with the examination, I might ask the patient some more questions that are thrown up by my examination. Throughout the process, I am happy to explain what my findings are. It is your body, you have the right to know. You should always ask the doctor what they are doing and what they think.

Too Much Disease, but Too Little Health

Professor Timothy Noakes,[1] an authority in sports medicine and sports science, who also happens to be a runner himself, in his thought-provoking book *Challenging Beliefs: Memoirs of a Career*, makes some interesting observations. Early on in his career, he understood that patients are best served by doctors who have first cured themselves of the doctors' disease—the pathological compulsion to cure. He goes on to add that we (doctors) know too much about disease but too little about health. We know everything about the limitations of the human body but not enough about its potentials. We are sometimes guilty of treating the disease and ignoring the patient.

In the current healthcare industry, starting from medical colleges, the focus is on the sick and the ill. They almost never look at normal, healthy human beings. The closest we got to normal was when we went to the dissection rooms, where it was rightly mentioned, 'where the dead teach the living'.

Think of your body as a computer. Till it is working well, there is no need to understand how it works, or that's what we assume. Yet, once it starts giving trouble, it helps immensely to know some very fundamental stuff about it; so the engineers don't take you for a ride—in this case my doctor colleagues.

The biggest problem that ails healthcare practitioners today is the 'if-I-don't-know-it-must-be-rubbish' syndrome. They also believe that whatever they specialize in is the solution for everything under the sun. Rather than getting into this 'ego' clash, their focus should be on getting you better, and help you lead a better life; a life where you are able to do justice to your body. This might, and usually does, involve knowledge of various fields out there, some of which could qualify as allopathic and some might not. They need to be open-minded, rather than have a tunnel vision.

Being Human

Dr Nanak Boparai, a friend from medical college, who is now a renowned paediatrician in the US, narrated an interesting but tragic story. A six-month-old baby had to undergo a life-saving surgery. Afterwards, there were all kinds of tubes going into her tiny body. Nanak was holding the baby in his hands. The surgeon peeped into the room and said, 'The kid looks great.' Nanak responded, 'She is dead.'

Most probably that surgeon only meant well but he was so busy between surgeries that he couldn't even look at the baby for a few seconds. Even if it was a complicated surgery with very low success rate, he had taken on the challenge. That child was his responsibility. He owed her a few seconds, post-surgery. Very unfortunate!

A physiotherapist had been treating a patient for back and hip pain for over six months. They had built up a good rapport. The elderly patient was dependant on the physiotherapist. One fine day, the physiotherapist decided to move on from that job. On being asked if she could have a conversation with the patient to explain her move, her response, without thinking even for a fraction of a second, was, 'I don't care.'

Being a physician or therapist of any kind simply isn't about being a good technician. It's about being human. There is no point if we all forget our human instincts and start acting like robots.

Dr Vert Mooney,[2] a distinguished orthopaedic surgeon who did groundbreaking work on conservative management of back pain, was of the opinion:

> We (doctors) have to be wary of the excessive enthusiasm for a belief system without supporting data. Sometimes we have to admit that the treatments advocated are only a current conceptual framework. We all have to be wary of belief in the religion of our experience and training, rather than the reality of what works and does not.

The 'if I don't know, it must be rubbish' attitude of experts is a huge problem in the healthcare fraternity. They don't even make an effort to learn or understand. That closed-mindedness and insecurity of specialists is not at all helpful for patients. It only confuses them further.

To add to that, Dr Michael Hutson, consultant musculoskeletal physician, Park Row Clinic, Nottingham, in his *Textbook of Musculoskeletal Medicine*[3] highlights something even more disturbing:

> A time consuming but potentially rewarding part of my work over the last 5–10 years has been to disabuse many patients of misconceptions regarding the nature of their back pain and to reverse the effects of its past mismanagement, instilled by 'conventional wisdom' of the medical profession over the last 30 or so years. These misconceptions so often arise from the discussion of 'crumbling spine', 'worn out discs', and 'arthritis' arising from X-ray (and now MRI as well) appearance, paying no heed to the findings of a competent musculoskeletal examination. Old habits die hard. A lot of my time goes doing the same.

Now, how do we handle the situation in the current scenario? Doctors might have a superiority complex, where we want to own all kinds of conditions and patients. It might be right in some medical conditions, but definitely not when it comes to pain. Even though it shouldn't be your problem, but it is. It's you who has the pain, so you need to understand and appreciate this.

Family doctors play a very important role in helping you with your pain, but then come along all these specialities: musculoskeletal medicine, orthopaedics, neurology, rheumatology, anaesthesiology, psychology, sports-exercise medicine and rehabilitation. To add to this, non-medical specialities like physiotherapy, osteopathy, chiropractors, yoga, Pilates, Alexander techniques and massages also have an important role in managing pain.

Some patients do claim that Ayurveda and homeopathy work as well. I don't want to comment on that as I don't know enough about them. However, it's important to know that homeopathy, which has got too much bad press because of some doctors calling it quackery, has far fewer side effects than allopathic medicines.

More than anything else, you need to understand that most lower back pains (as high as 98 per cent) don't need surgical intervention, at least not right away. You need to have a plan of action with the help of the doctors you consult. It should have three basic steps in the following order: conservative 'appropriate' proactive approach, 'interventional' approach (minimally invasive non-surgical: injections) and 'surgical' approach.

Conservative 'Appropriate' Proactive Approach

A lot of patients claim to have tried conservative treatment, which hasn't helped. The magic word here should be 'appropriate'. Sadly, in India today, a conservative approach to pain translates into either 'bed rest' or 'electrotherapy' at a physiotherapy clinic or rehabilitation department at a hospital. Neither are enough when it comes to managing pain appropriately. This book deals in detail with conservative pain management, as it can treat most people with pain. Even the ones who need the other two steps still need to undergo 'appropriate' conservative approach to have the best results. The specialities that should address this are musculoskeletal medicine, psychology, sports-exercise medicine, rehabilitation, rheumatology, anaesthesiology, orthopaedics, neurology, physiotherapy, osteopathy and chiropractors along with yoga, Pilates, Alexander techniques and massage.

In the film, *The Avengers*, there are several superheroes trying to save the world. They struggle to work as a team. The villain knows this weakness and exploits the situation well.

Similarly, it's fascinating to note that all these specialities in medicine have claimed ownership of 'pain management', when in fact they need to work together as a team to deal with the 'enemy'. Since a lot of specialities have laid claim to pain, there is great mistrust and misunderstanding amongst them. There can be no one single field that can do it on its own.

On a recent visit to one of the top corporate hospitals in Delhi, I saw a big poster announcing 'Institute of Musculoskeletal Sciences'. It mentioned the collective experience of the team: 15,000 joint replacements, 6,000 spine surgeries, 5,000 arthroscopic procedures, 2,000 paediatric orthopaedic surgeries, 1,000 foot and ankle surgeries and 1,000 hand surgeries. Even though more than 95 per cent of patients suffering from musculoskeletal conditions don't need surgeries, there was no mention of specialists who could address those conditions conservatively. Sadly, it's all about return on investment.

I have tried to 'educate' such set-ups on a holistic approach where the patient is at the centre of focus, but today's healthcare industry is simply too focused on themselves. Patients are just numbers, they just happen to be there.

I have actually given up on being part of the team of *Avengers*, all superheroes there. I am happy being Calvin from Calvin and Hobbes, a comic strip by American cartoonist Bill Watterson.

Specialities Taking 'Conservative' Route to Manage Back Pain

General practitioners, sports medicine doctors and musculoskeletal medicine doctors are the ones who tend to usually take a conservative approach to back pain. On their own they can't do much. They would need the help of allied health professionals like physiotherapists, chiropractors, osteopaths, acupuncturists, masseurs, yoga and Pilates instructors.

Physiotherapists

They are supposed to be the foot soldiers of back pain in the healthcare industry. They can address a majority of back pains that do not need surgical intervention. To become a physiotherapist/physical therapist, one must undergo a four-year bachelor/undergraduate course, which is a paramedical field. *Physiotherapist* comes from the words *physical* and *therapist*. In most parts of the world, the term used is physical therapy. It involves, or should involve, physical therapies including manual therapy, massage, mobilization and manipulations. In addition, it uses exercises to improve posture and muscle imbalances.

In India, most physiotherapists are poorly trained. It's not they but the system that is to be blamed. They end up only using modalities like ultrasound, interferential and laser treatments for all aches and pains, which medical research over the years hasn't shown to be very effective; definitely not in long-term and chronic conditions.

Although used in clinical practice for many years, current evidence-based clinical practice guidelines[4] do not endorse electrotherapy modalities (such as ultrasound, laser, interferential) in the management of lower back pain, due to lack of evidence of effects on clinically relevant outcomes. Instead, patients with subacute lower back pain should be advised to stay active and referred for prescribed analgesia if necessary. For chronic lower back pain, helpful interventions include short-term use of medication/manipulation/ acupuncture, supervised exercise therapy, cognitive behavioural therapy and multidisciplinary treatment.

If you've had back pain for a while and your back has been inactive for a long time, it's important to undergo a rehabilitation programme under supervision. It needs to involve the three pillars of fitness and rehabilitation— strengthening, stretching and cardiovascular activity. None of the three can replace the other ones. Neither gym instructors nor most physiotherapists are equipped to cater to this when you have pain.

My simple advice is that if a physiotherapist doesn't touch your back or the part that is painful, leave alone a full musculoskeletal examination, you are wasting your time. Good physiotherapists will understand the underlying problem. They will make you do exercises under supervision and make an exercise plan to cater to your muscle imbalances to improve your posture, so that your body is able to cater to its own needs.

Spinal Manipulations (Chiropractors, Osteopaths, Physiotherapists)

There is no formal training in India for either osteopathy or chiropractic, but both are popular for the treatment of back pain in the West. Both are a combination of bone-setters and medical doctors who have undergone formal training unlike bone-setters found in India who are mostly full-time cobblers and part time bone-setters. Osteopaths and chiropractors are good at taking detailed history of the patient and doing a thorough musculoskeletal examination.

Please note, of late, in India it's become fashionable for physiotherapists to do a weekend course in osteopathy or chiropractic techniques and then call themselves either osteopaths or chiropractors. These short courses will not suffice for four years of training in either of the fields. I would be weary of such characters.

Good osteopaths and chiropractors are well trained in posture assessment and correction through education and treatment. They then are well equipped to come up with a functional diagnosis and look beyond the conventional diagnosis. Their objective is to help you use your body optimally. They can perform manipulations and mobilizations that range from gentle soft tissue release and therapeutic massages, to bone articulations, to manipulations of joints.

Chiropractors, osteopaths and physiotherapists should be well trained in manual therapy, and use spinal manipulations to diagnose, treat and prevent neuro musculoskeletal conditions, especially aches and pains. Manual therapy (therapeutic massage, joint adjustments, manipulations and subluxations) works wonders for some at times, but not for all, all the time. The therapists should be able to choose their patients carefully, and not just perform the manipulation on everyone because they've been trained in it. Traditionally, chiropractors tend to do more joint adjustments as compared to osteopaths who focus a bit more on lifestyle. Physiotherapists, tend to use more of electrotherapeutic modalities.[5]

You must remember that these manual therapeutic techniques will bring about only a short-term change. It's good for now, but you need to do more. Unless you combine it with a better lifestyle, posture, breathing, attitude and exercise schedule, any positive change is not going to last. Good therapists, no matter from which stream, tend not to focus merely on the problem area as presented by their patient, but consider contributions from anatomically distant parts of the musculoskeletal system, the mind and social influences when trying to understand a patient's problem and producing a management plan.

I am a trained medical osteopath who practices manipulation when needed, and I also train physiotherapists in spinal manipulation. It's simply not about being biased. However, denial is not helpful either. We need to be honest with ourselves about the situation and address it appropriately.

Case: Ramesh Mohan (name changed), thirty-two years old

In 2005, Ramesh Mohan, a thirty-two-year-old unemployed gentleman, who had been suffering from upper back and chest pain for over a year, consulted me at a hospital in Delhi while I was visiting from London. He had gone to various doctors who had ruled out all serious conditions including cardiac diseases, since all tests had turned out to be normal. When I saw him, he was on a waiting list to be operated for his spine. I was only supposed to examine him, as a demonstration to the physiotherapists of that department.

Mohan was not going to fall for some voodoo or placebo. He had severe pain which had messed up his professional and personal life. He had been fired from his job as he was always complaining of pain and was not productive at all. While examining him, I found a bit of restriction in his upper back (mid-thoracic spine). In passing, I articulated (a manual therapy technique) his upper back and gave him some basic exercises.

When I met him a week later, a day before he was to be operated, his pain had gone. It was no magic. It was just that no one had examined his back properly and given him an appropriate exercise programme. The surgeon was annoyed with me. Leave alone a call appreciating the help, he began to talk poorly about me in medical circles.

I got to know later that the patient had been convinced by the surgeon that for long-term relief, he needed surgery. I am not sure for what since his MRI was normal too. The poor fellow did undergo surgery. Isn't this a criminal offence? So much for the noble profession!

Acupuncture

Acupuncture is again one of those treatment modalities that has got mixed reviews as far as research evidence goes. Some patients get an amazing response, but some don't respond as well. As far as I am concerned, the big positive in its favour is it doesn't have any side effects.

I personally have had very good results with acupuncture in calming down pain.

Case: Ved Prakash Chauhan, fifty-four years old

Sixteen years ago, a fifty-four-year-old patient had been having severe lower back pain going down his right leg for over six months. He carried his MRIs with him which showed disc bulge at two levels in the lower back (lumbar 4/5, lumbar 5, Sacral 1) along with degenerative changes. He had consulted three or four orthopaedic surgeons before seeing me. All but one had suggested surgery. I was pretty much his last resort before he considered surgery seriously.

I had been undergoing tutelage in medical acupuncture after my medical degree because I found myself very keen in pain but found traditional treatments not as useful. I was by no means a believer in acupuncture but had seen some patients with lower back pain get remarkably better with it. I took up Chauhan's case because I was clear about one thing, maybe I couldn't make him better, but I was not going to make him worse. No harm in exhausting all conservative approaches before he was to undergo the surgery.

He underwent eighteen sessions with me in about a month and by the end of it his pain had almost disappeared. Could I explain why that happened. No. Did I do some magic? Definitely not. Looking back at it now, I realize that I was very confident during the consultations and during treatment sessions. I was confident because I had witnessed very high success rates with acupuncture in lower back pain cases.

My touch wasn't very confident but it was enough to make Chauhan feel confident enough in whatever I was doing. I had relaxed his lower back muscles through acupuncture. I gave him some very gentle exercises.

Acupuncture worked in this case. Since then I have trained in dry needling in London. I don't use it all the time but have trained my staff over the last decade in India. At times, it works wonderfully well but there are times when it just hasn't worked.

Massage

In cases of severe pain, I highly recommend not to experiment. Most masseurs are not trained to address pain, so it is best not to risk it. Not for now, at least.

On the other hand, it's important to also keep in mind that 'touch' is a very powerful tool. Even a very light touch is known to give relief. If you are not sure but still want to get a massage done, it is best to go for light massages. It simply calms down the muscles involved.

Yoga and Pilates

Both yoga and Pilates have a role in back pain but I would advise against either if you have severe pain. The simple reason being that most teachers and trainers in both these fields are not trained enough to deal with pain.

I have seen enough cases where the trainer or teacher has excitedly taken on the challenge of treating back pain using either yoga or Pilates without having enough knowledge to do the same. They have ended up making simple back pain cases far worse than they started with.

One must locate a good instructor. Even in places like New York, London, Berlin and Barcelona, there are very few good instructors who are comfortable with managing pain.

With due respect to both fields, in the long-term they still do not provide enough strengthening. Again, I am trained in both and clearly know the limitations in the current scenario. I urge trainers and therapists not to treat the fields they are trained in like a religion. Think sensibly.

Non-Steroidal Anti-Inflammatory Drugs (NSAIDs)

NSAIDS or any other over-the-counter medications for pain should be used with caution.[6]

Non-steroidal anti-inflammatory drugs (NSAIDs) are frequently used to treat moderate acute pain. They are not usually required after the cause of the acute pain has been addressed. Treatment should be reassessed if the acute pain is ongoing and not resolved within two weeks. Better to see a specialist than playing one.

Oral NSAIDs have considerable cardiovascular, gastrointestinal and kidney function risks. They should not be recommended without consideration of the patient's additional diseases or conditions; particularly in older people, people with kidney disease, those with a history of peptic ulcer disease, hypertension or heart failure.

Older people should use the lowest possible dose of an oral NSAID, for the shortest duration possible and multiple NSAIDs should not be taken at the same time. The effectiveness of long-term oral NSAID treatment should be routinely assessed against the individual patient's management plan. If possible, the total dose should be reduced or ceased.

Products containing a low dose (less than 12 mg) of codeine per tablet combined with another analgesic medicine are available without a prescription and are commonly recommended for the treatment of mild to moderate pain.[7]

Codeine is converted to morphine in the body to work. The extent of this metabolism depends on each individual's pharmacogenetics, which are not readily known and this highly varies between individuals.

There is evidence that doses of codeine, less than 30 mg every 6 hours, are no more effective than paracetamol or an NSAID alone. Therefore, combination products that contain low-dose codeine should not be recommended for mild to moderate pain. If used, their effectiveness should be assessed within 48 hours. If symptoms persist, the product should be ceased and the patient referred for further assessment.

Codeine can lead to constipation, nausea, vomiting, bloating and abdominal pain. Any of these symptoms can impact the quality of life.

'Interventional' Approach

The 'interventional' approach to pain is managed by anaesthesiologists who use oral medications and injections to address pain. A lot of advancement has happened in this field in the recent past. This works very well with the 'appropriate', conservative approach. At times, the patient needs the interventional procedure to be done first, so that it's easier to work with the 'proactive' part of the 'appropriate' conservative approach. At other times, it is recommended after having attempted it for some time, but not getting the desired results.

Anaesthesiologists

Anaesthesiology is a postgraduate (MD) degree after MBBS. Traditionally, their role has been to anaesthetize the patient for a surgery, so that the patient doesn't experience pain. It is only recently in India that they have started running 'pain clinics'. Here, the anaesthesiologists look to manage pain using injections and other interventional approaches. They have an important role in managing back pain, more so when combined with a holistic view of pain and the human body.

It's only after you've exhausted conservative modalities, both passive and active, would I suggest injections and/or surgeries—unless of course it is an emergency.

Nerve root block is a kind of an injection procedure that targets irritated nerves. Injections usually given for back pain contain steroids. This has unnecessarily got a lot of negative reviews. Steroids are present in the human body and play an important role in healing and immunity. In injections, small doses are given and that too in a localized way. There is a good reason for it being done. They are very safe procedures.

Rheumatologists

Sometimes back pain can occur because of conditions that are addressed well by rheumatologists. They study rheumatology as a super-speciality after MBBS and MD or as special interest as part of MD. Because of their training, their approach is to take a medical route to address the problem at hand. They could use modalities such as injections, besides medicines.

The 'Surgical' Approach

Most surgeries that are needed in back pain cases are elective surgeries, if at all. You should definitely undergo the first step of 'appropriate' proactive conservative management before surgery. You also need to undergo appropriate rehabilitation. The exercise programme usually prescribed after surgery is just not enough. There needs to be a graded programme, which will push your body appropriately.

When Should You Consider Surgery?

If your lower back pain hasn't responded to conservative management, especially a proactive multidisciplinary approach, or a minimally invasive intervention such as injections, and has affected your quality of life markedly, it is important to consider surgery. Different surgical procedures that can be done depending on the cause are: removing a herniated disc, widening the space around the spinal cord and fusing two or more spinal vertebrae together.

As mentioned earlier, emergency surgery is very rarely needed in case of back pain. However, if you have any of the following, please do get to the hospital right away just to rule out any serious cause. It's not meant to scare you, but to make you aware. By definition, emergency comes along unannounced.

1. Sudden loss of sensation in one or both legs, with or without loss of sensation in the buttock region.
2. Sudden loss of control of bowel and bladder movements. You could feel as if you are not in control. There is dribbling even after you have finished urinating.
3. Sudden weakness of one or both legs, which is not because of just pain.
4. Pain while passing urine.

Specialities Taking Surgical Route to Manage Back Pain

Orthopaedic Surgeons

They end up being the first line of defence for back pain. In principle, it is not a bad choice. They know the skeletal system very well. So, if they look at you as a human being rather than a painful body part, that's the doctor you need.

Unfortunately, very similar to the shortage of general physicians because of demand and supply imbalances, there are also now fewer general orthopaedicians. They are turning into specialists that deal with joint replacements, particular body parts, etc. In addition to that, you need to understand that a surgeon is trained to operate, that's what they are good at. In their training years all they have seen is that patients do benefit immensely from surgery.

The issue is that a majority of patients, who could have become better without surgeries, are advised surgery. None of us like to be operated on. When a patient refuses surgery, the next best option for the orthopaedician is to put him on medication to calm the pain. Without realizing, the patient gets addicted to them. They also end up advising the patient to rest longer than he should.

So, orthopaedic surgeons are good for advice on back pain, but I would suggest to look for the ones who are more conservative rather than trigger-happy.

Neurosurgeons or Neurologists

It's the neuro musculoskeletal system that we are dealing with. Neurosurgeons and neurologists have a definite role in back pain and other pain cases. Neurosurgery is generally a super-speciality you do after doing general surgery. During their training, they see a lot more general cases of all kinds, not only of a specific kind. This makes them a little more open-minded about the approach taken for back pain.

What Do People Want in a Good Doctor?

'What do you expect your doctor to be like?' I posed this question on social media.

To be a 'good attentive listener' was by far the commonest feature that respondents were looking for. He or she should form an opinion only after hearing the patient out.

This was closely followed by a lot of other features like a good doctor should be caring, filled with empathy, dedicated, responsive, who doesn't order unnecessary tests and diagnoses based on the patient's story and examination, definitely not surgeries when there is no need. He or she should definitely be confident and explain things clearly. He should take decisions with the patient rather than for him or her. What was fascinating for me was that not even one respondent was interested in the number of degrees the doctors had or which college the doctors had attended or how big a hospital they worked in.

Of course, doctors need to be competent but these soft skills mentioned above are the ones that make the doctors humans, especially when dealing with pain. They aren't simply supposed to be technicians fixing a broken car or a machine.

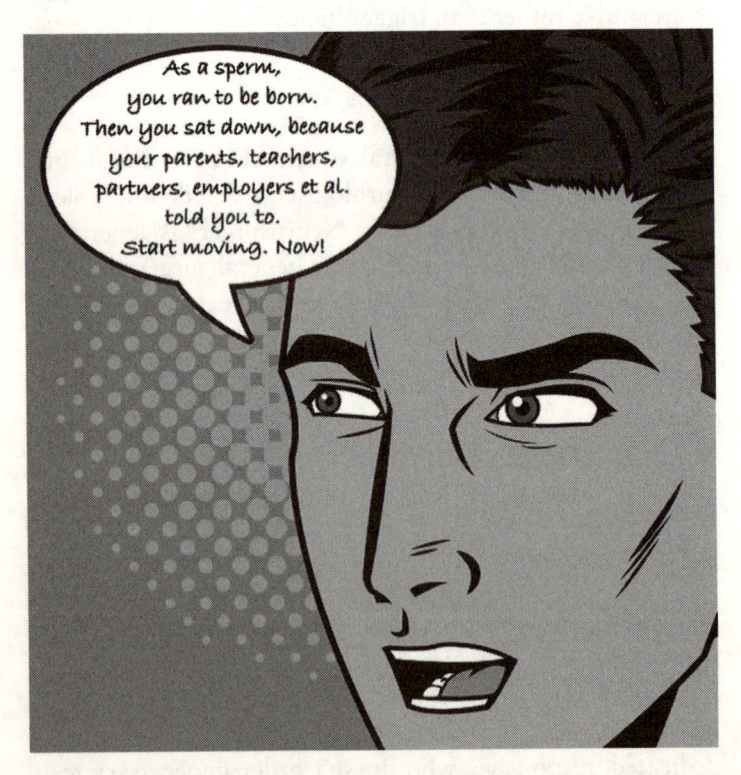

4

TESTS AND INVESTIGATIONS

'Unlike some other areas of medicine, musculoskeletal conditions often produce symptoms and signs that render a diagnosis possible without further investigation. With a thorough, logical history and clinical examination, a diagnosis should be possible in the majority of musculoskeletal cases. In order to be able to commence treatment promptly and also to avoid unnecessary expense and use of resources, over-investigation is to be avoided.'[1]

A couple of things have been highlighted in the above statement. First, the role of investigations in back pain is limited as compared to other areas of medicine. History and clinical examinations are a lot more important. Second, treating back pain is more of an art than a science.

Depending only on latest high-tech investigations to diagnose and then base the treatment on these findings just doesn't work in the case of back pain. This is sadly being practised by doctors today. We are supposed to be treating you, rather than your reports alone.

What then is the role of investigations in treating back pain?

a. To confirm the diagnosis when in doubt.
b. To assess the degree of severity and see if the treatment needs to change.
c. To confirm or rule out serious diseases (cancer, fracture, tuberculosis and so on) that might also cause back pain. If they are detected, the treatment needs to change accordingly.
d. Some patients might associate the most serious condition with their back pain. Conducting investigations reassures the patients and helps them move on from the disease.

Investigations for back pain are broadly divided into three categories:

a. Imaging: X-ray, CT scan, MRI, myelography, discography, isotope bone scan, ultrasound
b. Blood tests: Full blood count (FBC), erythrocyte sedimentation rate (ESR), C-reactive protein (CRP)
c. Other tests: Electromyography (EMG)

Imaging

Several patients in India mistake investigations (tests) for therapeutic (treatment) tools, so they get them done without the advice from a doctor or therapist. They do that to bypass doctors. Patients get this perception from the doctors they go to. This has led to patients undergoing unnecessary tests.

About 80–90 per cent of back pain that is reported can be categorized as non-specific, mechanical lower back pain. The commonest findings in this are abnormal muscle function, muscle imbalances and postural problems, which cannot be shown by conventional and commonly used imaging investigations including X-ray, MRI, CT and so on, or even joint blocks and discography.

Even though, these investigations are important to obtain information, they are being performed too often and too soon into the treatment. This has led to the mismanagement of back pain. More often than not, some abnormality shows up, which has nothing to do with the pain; but the patient and the doctor use it to justify the back pain and opt for treatment, accordingly.

The world over, top medical societies and associations[2], recommend that patients with non-specific lower back pain should not get imaging done unless a serious cause like cancer or infection is suspected. This is usually not the case.

The imaging investigations done for back pain are generally very sensitive. They pick up things that aren't even bothering the patients. Remember the time (if you rode bicycles to school) when the tyre of the bicycle would get punctured and you had to take it to a repair shop? The shopkeeper would tell you multiple other places where the tyre was about to get punctured, but those punctures never happened. You were made to take 'precautionary measures' to address the 'potential puncture' sites only because that was the business model that worked perfectly well for the bicycle repair shop. Similarly, medical investigations are simply serving the healthcare 'workshops'.

In 1993, Dr Alf Nachemson[3] said, 'During the last decade, we have had an enormous increase in imaging and surgical technology. CT, MRI, etc., demonstrate anatomic changes which often have no importance at all for the patient's pain.' More than two decades later, both patients and doctors are still doing what Dr Nachemson pointed out.

Dr Vert Mooney[4], a renowned orthopaedic surgeon and a pioneer in using exercises for lower back pain, said:

> We (doctors) are all treating disordered human anatomy and function of some type. Thus, the reasonable baseline of understanding anatomic deviation has to be the starting point of the discussion. Some of this is measurable by radiography (X-ray) and physical examination, but most of the functional disorders under consideration are not truly measurable, such as muscle spasms, tenderness, or induration. We (doctors) all know about these phenomena, but the significance and severity of palpatory finding is varied. On the other hand, plain radiographs (X-ray) and MRIs may even be misleading in their attempt to supply objective evidence of skeletal and articular abnormality.

There is also a tendency amongst doctors, when they don't find anything wrong in imaging investigations, to suggest that there is a psychological cause for back pain. Of course, there always is, but it's never the sole reason.

X-rays

> Love is a lot like a backache, it doesn't show up on X-rays, but you know it's there.
>
> —George Burns (1896–1996)

X-rays have been around since 1895 when they were discovered by Roentgen. It was American physiologist Walter Bradford Cannon who realized their medical application.

Today, the commonest investigation requested for back pain is an X-ray. It is a very affordable investigation, which has probably led to it being overused as an investigative tool, even when it doesn't play an important role. All 'lower back pain management' guidelines by international medical bodies globally have questioned the use of X-rays to investigate lower back pain, but doctors continue to prescribe them.

What to Expect?

a. You don't need to fast for a back X-ray.
b. You'll be asked to remove your jewellery or any other metal items. You might be asked to wear a gown for the X-ray.
c. You might be asked to lie down on a table and then the X-ray will be done. You might be asked to lie in different positions to get different views of your spine.
d. Normally, it should take you no more than 10 minutes for the whole procedure.

X-rays have a role in back pain when there is a bony pathology:

a. Vertebral fracture and collapse
b. Scoliosis and spondylosis/spondylolisthesis
c. Dislocation
d. Arthritic changes
e. Suspected metastasis (spreading) of cancer
f. Chronic disease such as tuberculosis

There is good reason to markedly reduce the use of X-rays.

a. Any of the bony pathologies mentioned above are very infrequent to be a cause for back pain—as little as 1 per cent of all back pains.
b. Circumstantial evidence of soft tissue damage can also be picked on an X-ray, like reduced space between two vertebrae (spine bones), which is suggestive of a disc bulge. Most people, who have a disc bulge, don't have back pain. History and examination becomes very important to determine if the disc bulge is the cause of the pain. In any case, X-rays don't help in the case of disc bulges. MRIs need to be done to confirm a suspected disc bulge, if at all.
c. Most findings on X-rays don't correlate with back pain complaints. It's been very commonly observed that people whose lower back X-rays show degenerative changes very often don't have any back pain. Sometimes the reverse is possible too. A person could have severe back pain, but the X-ray would be completely normal. It becomes very important to rely on clinical examination rather than simply on X-rays. When X-rays are done in a rush, both patient and doctor try to justify the X-ray findings.
d. The body is exposed to radiations while undergoing lumbar spine, pelvis or hip X-rays. This increases the risk of developing cancers of different kinds.
e. Avoid lumbar spine, pelvis and hip X-rays for young children and pregnant ladies even though the radiations emitted are safe for the foetus. It's more precautionary than anything else. It should be done for pregnant women only if there are unavoidable circumstances. Let your doctor decide that for you.
f. The National Institute for Health and Care Excellence (NICE)[5] guidelines state: For the management of non-specific lower back pain, an X-ray of the lumbar spine is not required.

MRI (Magnetic Resonance Imaging)

Magnetic Resonance Imaging (MRI) scan is an investigation of choice for back pain, especially when a disc or nerve is suspected to be the culprit.

MRIs became popular in the 1980s in the West and by the 1990s, MRI centres mushroomed everywhere because of their medical application. It is a relatively expensive investigation, with no exposure to any radiation. This makes it a safer investigation than the cheaper, easily available X-rays.

MRI has been a major breakthrough in medicine and it has changed the way we look at the human body and diseases. For better or worse, it has also changed how lower back pain is looked at, both by patients and doctors. For the slightest of issues, patients themselves get MRIs done. They want to see what has gone wrong in their body that is causing them that discomfort or pain. In any case, most doctors ask for an MRI.

MRI gives a detailed view of the interior of the body but it is exactly like a still photograph. It is informative but doesn't tell you a thing about the background and its context. It is simply an abstract. MRIs have to be viewed with the detailed history of the patient. As Dr Harsh Mahajan, one of the top radiologist in Delhi, points out, 'Treat the patient, not the MRI.'

MRI is only supposed to help the doctors come to a conclusion along with detailed history and physical examination. Unfortunately, a lot of doctors out there only treat the MRIs. I have a question for these colleagues: Why operate? Just take an eraser and rub whatever you don't like in the MRI. But please don't try to treat the human body that you haven't even seen. A detailed history and thorough physical examination give me a lot more than an MRI in isolation.

'Structural changes on MRI are very common even at an early age; they correlate poorly with pain and disability, demonstrating that lower back pain is poorly related to structural pathology. Education is an important intervention. Reassuring people that LBP [lower back pain] is rarely linked to structural damage, that pain does not equal harm and that their back is structurally sound (even if painful) can reduce fear, catastrophizing and disability.'[6]

I ask my patients to get an MRI when the findings could possibly change my plan of action and when I am looking at referring a patient for surgery. NICE guidelines[7] are even stricter and suggest that an MRI scan for non-specific lower back pain should be done only if spinal fusion is being considered.

As NICE guidelines[8] suggest, MRI is also recommended when suspecting serious medical conditions such as spinal malignancy, infection, fracture, cauda equina syndrome or ankylosing spondylitis or another inflammatory disorder.

What to Expect?

a. MRI scan machines are tubes; patients have to lie inside these during a scan.
b. The scanner applies a strong magnetic field across body tissues. Constant turning on and off of the magnetic field causes a lot of noise in the tube which is not very comfortable for some patients.
c. Patients need to lie still in the tube for 20–40 minutes. Patients might feel claustrophobic or restless inside the tube.
d. Nowadays open MRI scanners are available but are more expensive and not easily available. There is also a compromise on the quality of scans.

Role of MRI Scans

a. Since there is no radiation in MRI, they are considered safer than X-rays and CT scans.
b. When disc or nerve root pathology is suspected, MRI scans are the imaging investigation of choice.
c. MRIs are also investigation of choice in suspected infections and tumours.
d. If back pain persists for long or surgery is being considered, MRI is definitely advised.

When Not to Opt for an MRI Scan

a. MRIs are not to be done in case of pacemakers, defibrillators and metal bodies in the eyes, aneurysm clips in the brain and shunts in the central nervous system (CNS).
b. To be avoided in the first trimester during pregnancy.
c. To be avoided by patients with any metal implants or prosthesis, cochlear implants or artificial heart valve.

There is a good reason to markedly reduce the usage of MRIs. Way too many of them are being done. In 2011 and 2012 respectively, MRIs were the seventh and eighth 'most-shopped' healthcare service by patients.[9]

Studies[10] have shown that even amongst patients not having any back pain, 83 per cent had moderate to severe desiccation of one or more discs, 64 per cent had one or more bulging discs, 56 per cent had loss of disc height, 32 per cent had at least one disc protrusion and 6 per cent had one or more disc extrusions.

The doctors, intentionally or unintentionally, based on the MRI findings mentioned above, suggest procedures like injections and surgeries, which are often not needed. Even if these procedures are needed, they are done too soon.

CT Scans

Computed Tomography (CT) Scans are done when MRIs can't be done because of a metal implant or pacemaker. As the name suggests, CT scans are multiple X-ray images that are computed to give two-dimensional and three-dimensional images, showing both bones and soft tissues.

What to Expect?

a. Patients need to lie down for 20–30 minutes.
b. Since there is no tunnel, like in MRI, claustrophobic patients can opt for a CT scan as an alternative investigation.

Role of CT Scans

a. CT scans are important when MRIs can't be done, e.g., in metal implants or pacemakers.
b. As compared to MRIs, which are better at picking soft tissue abnormalities, CT scans are better at picking bone abnormalities.

There are reasons to markedly reduce the usage of CT scans.

a. There is some exposure to radiation, as is the case with X-rays; so it should only be done after careful consideration.
b. CT scans should be avoided in pregnancy and among children.
c. Contrast dye used during the procedure may cause temporary kidney damage, the risk of which is higher in pre-existing kidney disease or infection.

Myelography

Myelography used to be the investigation of choice till MRI came along. A dye is injected into the spinal canal to highlight it, the spinal cord and the spinal nerves. It is a longer procedure than MRI, and because it is invasive, it can be uncomfortable with some side effects as well.

Role of Myelography

a. Myelography is suggested when MRI is not possible.
b. Some studies show that spinal canal narrowing[11] and nerve compression[12] are not seen properly in MRI scans as compared to myelography.

Discography

Discography is not done very frequently in cases of back pain. It becomes important before a surgical procedure like fusion of vertebrae because of degenerated disc(s) in between, leading to instability between corresponding vertebrae. As mentioned above, MRI and X-ray could show if there is any damage to the disc along with instability, but it is not necessary that these are the reasons for the pain. Discography could help in confirming if the intervertebral disc is responsible for the pain.

What to Expect?

a. A dye is injected into the centre of the disc. This would lead to increase in pressure in the disc.
b. If this elicits more pain than what the patient usually experiences, the disc is suspected to be the culprit.
c. In such cases, ozone nucleolysis and fusion could help in getting rid of the pain.

d. As it is an invasive procedure, there will be a higher risk of side effects as compared to X-rays, MRIs and CT scans. There could be nerve damage and serious infection of disc (discitis).

Role of Discography

Discography might play a role in taking the final decision on fusion surgery. However, it is not a foolproof investigation:

a. There is a high chance of discography suggesting that the pain is coming from the disc when that's not really the case.
b. For this reason, discography should be saved as a last resort and strictly done only on the advice of the surgeon who is suggesting fusion.

Isotope Bone Scan

A radioactive substance is injected that shows the blood flow and the bone turnover. Bone scans are done when osteoarthritis, fractures, spread (metastasis) of cancer and infections are suspected but X-rays have not shown anything conclusive. The ionizing radiations emitted are higher than in X-rays, so bone scans should be done only when there is a real need.

Role of Bone Scans

a. Might be useful to see the spread of cancer.

Ultrasound

In ultrasound, high frequency sound waves are passed through body tissues to demonstrate the appearance of normal and abnormal muscles, tendons and tendon sheaths. Since ultrasound doesn't use any ionizing radiation, it is safe for pregnant women and young children.

Ultrasound has been used to measure the activity of core stability muscles (abdominal and back), which cause lower back pain. Ultrasound might have an important role in the measurement of joint laxity (looseness) too, which have also been associated with lower back pain.[13]

The biggest negative about ultrasound is that the results are very dependent on the skill of the user. It takes a while to master the technique. Since it is a relatively cheaper investigation, a lot of doctors and hospitals don't prescribe it.

Blood Tests in Back Pain

Blood tests are easily available and usually not very expensive. They are prescribed in back pain if infection, cancer or other inflammatory conditions (rheumatoid arthritis, etc.) are suspected.

Full blood count (FBC), erythrocyte sedimentation rate (ESR) and C-reactive protein (CRP) are usually enough in back pain cases. If infection or inflammation is suspected, ESR and CRP play a role. For patients who are suspected to be suffering from rheumatoid arthritis, rheumatoid factor (RF) and anti-cyclic citrullinated peptide (anti-CCP) are important blood tests. For those with ankylosing spondylitis, human leukocyte antigen (HLA-B27) is recommended.

Specialized Nerve Tests

As mentioned earlier, the lowest part of the brain continues as spinal cord in the spinal canal. These nerves are very similar to electric wires. The brain and spinal cord send electrical signals through nerves to different muscles. If there is a disturbance in these nerves, whether it is by physical compression or chemical irritation, it disturbs the electrical signals.

Electromyography (EMG)

EMG detects the electricity generated by muscle cells when electric currents come to them through the corresponding nerves. There can be an abnormality in the spinal cord, nerves or the muscles that are connected to corresponding nerves. EMG can detect abnormal muscles.

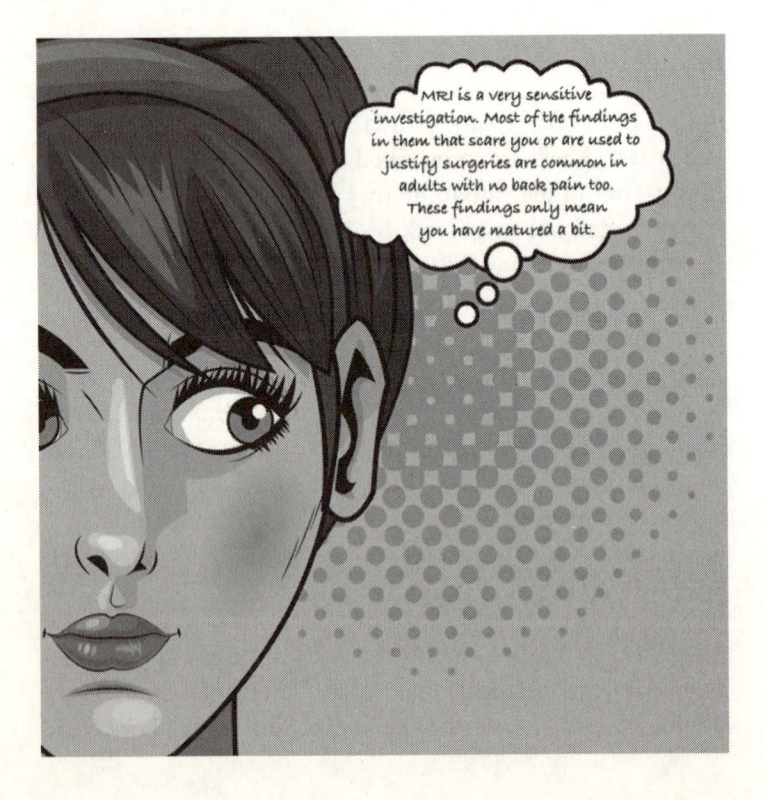

MRI is a very sensitive investigation. Most of the findings in them that scare you or are used to justify surgeries are common in adults with no back pain too. These findings only mean you have matured a bit.

5

COMMON DIAGNOSIS: CAUSES OF BACK PAIN

A majority of pains can be addressed by basic advice given in this book. Before I go on, it is important for you to understand and appreciate the fact that the whole body of yours needs to be treated, and not just your back.

Most conditions found during investigations could simply be coincidental or an effect of something else, not a cause in itself. If at all, it's only sometimes the cause.

I would always think of the commonest causes first, and not the rarest ones. This book is majorly dedicated to the commonest causes of back pain.

Simple Back Pain

In 90 per cent of back pain, there is no obvious reason for the pain. The technical term that is used is non-specific low back pains, which is self-explanatory. In these cases, most modern investigations are not able to find any abnormality. At times MRIs find abnormalities when there is no back pain, but the reverse is true as well. Most doctors and therapists end up blaming the patient for the pain and say it's a psychological or psychosomatic problem. It's all in their head.

Of course it's in the mind, everything is, but it's not the only thing.

In these cases, a detailed history and physical examination give a lot more information than high-tech investigations. The best way forward is to combine the art of medicine with the science of it.

I like to use the term *dysfunction* for common back pain, which is simply an abnormal function of muscles and tendons (muscle spasm and strain, muscle tension, muscle imbalance), ligaments (ligament sprain), fascia (myofascial restrictions) and joints (joint instability and joint restriction). This is a term commonly used in osteopathy. I tend to use it even more loosely. After the age of three or so, all of us start abusing our bodies more and more by increasingly doing activities that are unnatural to us, like sitting on chairs, wearing shoes, using computers and other gizmos. All of these keep accumulating and soon enough lead to gross muscle imbalances, which further lead to poor posture and other unhealthy habits. Early on in life age is in your favour, so it doesn't bother you much. But soon enough, done repeatedly, the change is permanent. This leads to underlying pain all the time.

Soon enough, you forget to breathe and move properly. From being naturally functional, you are now dysfunctional. All pains have a physical and psychological component that feed off each other. In addition, other contributors make sure you have a bad back and health, sooner than you had bargained for.

There is usually no single cause for pain but a lot of small factors that accumulate to cause it. Usually, it is the most insignificant movement that could bring on an attack of severe back pain. It's pretty much like the proverbial last straw that broke the camel's back.

Somatic dysfunction, what I simply like to call dysfunction, is a diagnosis that you would think some looney like me would come up with. In the Western world, it's not that rare to hear it. It might surprise you that this is actually recognized as a valid diagnostic term in the International Classification of Disease since 1972.

I'm not going into further details with this as enough has been covered on it in the book. Simply put, we were born to move, or we ran like hell to be born (do you recall being that tiny little sperm). Some would argue it was a race, but I think it was a very well-orchestrated run.

The commonest findings on physical examination in cases of non-specific low back pain are abnormal muscle function, muscle imbalances and poor posture. Over a period of time, these abnormal muscle functions lead to pathologies (abnormalities) including disc bulge and tear.

But people, both medics and non-medics, are under the impression that disc bulge is the commonest reason for back pain. In actual fact, that's only a cause in less than 5 per cent of lower back pain cases.

Non-specific mechanical lower back pain (cause for 80–90 per cent of all back aches) doesn't show up on the common investigations (X-ray, MRI, CT scan, etc.) or even on invasive investigations like joint blocks and discography, but most patients rush to get them even after two days of back pain. It's because some doctors do the same. Patients believe that doctors would anyway ask for these investigations, so might as well get them beforehand.

A thorough history (consultation) and physical examination is important for relieving anxiety about the consequences of pain and sufficient for identifying the patients who should be referred to another specialist for examination and treatment (eg., due to severe infection, specific rheumatic disease, suspected cancer, or other serious conditions).[1]

Even if there is a clear-cut diagnosis, like the ones mentioned below, you need to know that there could be underlying dysfunction which shouldn't be ignored. As soon as that is addressed, along with the multidisciplinary approach, even the pathologists start behaving a lot better. They have a better support system to rely on. In any case, most have happened because you ignored all the signs of dysfunction all these years. In our eagerness to treat the *disease*, we are only causing an effect with trying to remove the 'dis' and getting you at 'ease'.

Disc Bulges or Tears

Bulges and tears (20–40 years) and degeneration changes in discs and or facet joints (40–60 years) are a very distant, second commonest cause of lower back pain depending on your age. They are over-diagnosed by my doctor colleagues because all our medical books somehow can't understand the functioning of the back, or the lack of it. Unless there is pathology, it goes off radar.

As mentioned earlier, having a bad posture with poor body usage, exposes your lower back to high stress that can then lead to the above three conditions. It's very crucial to remember that as many as two-thirds of the population has been found to have a disc bulge without any symptoms.[2] MRI detects the disc bulge, but we need to see both clinical findings on physical examination and MRI findings together. If your disc bulge is asymptomatic and the pain is coming from somewhere else, we need to focus on that.

Sometimes there is an annular tear in the disc because of repeated stress, thanks to poor body usage and posture. This causes chemical irritation of the nerve and other tissues at that level.

Mechanical Lower Back Pain with Neurogenic Leg Pain

Of all back pains, 7–10 per cent lead to pain going down the leg. Nerve from a particular level of the spine, when irritated or injured, would cause pain going down the leg in a particular pattern. This happens when a nerve is irritated or compressed somewhere along its path. It could happen because of the corresponding bulging disc, bony changes limiting the foramen (opening) through which the nerve exits the vertebral column, or it could be a taut piriformis muscle (piriformis syndrome), a muscle in the buttock region that compresses the sciatic nerve.

Intervertebral Disc Herniation

This is also thought to be the most common cause of pain coming from the back, going down the leg. Intervertebral disc herniation can cause lower back pain, leg pain or both. Sometimes leg pain can be present without any back pain. The herniated disc is compressing the spinal cord or corresponding nerves exiting the foramina. Depending on which disc compresses a spinal nerve, the pain will radiate accordingly down the leg.

But contrary to popular beliefs, pain down the leg is not always because of the nerve being affected. It can happen because of a certain muscle not functioning properly, as discussed below.

Myofascial Pain[3]

This is the most common reason for pain radiating down the leg but is under-diagnosed. In this, a corresponding muscle is usually not functioning well because of muscle imbalances and poor posture.

Each muscle is comprised of individual bands of muscle tissues lying parallel to one another. These bands work together when muscles contract. When muscles stay in that abnormal contracted position because of a muscular strain, trauma or poor posture accompanied with bad habits, it results in 'taut bands'. A 'trigger point' is located in this taut band. This taut band is like a microspasm, a spasm of an individual band of the muscle. Besides causing pain where the taut band is, a trigger point can cause predictable referred pain pattern that is specific to that muscle. It usually doesn't go down all the way.

Degenerative Changes in Discs or Facet Joints

Again this is a diagnosis that is over-reported and a lot of misinformation is spread by health professionals. Using the wrong terminologies and talking about it carelessly to the patient (you) can only have a long-term, at times permanent, damage.

Degenerative changes in the spine have been blamed for most cases of back pain. As we age, there are going to be some natural changes, some would have more, some would have less. Yet, when this information is shared with a person having pain, it can have catastrophic effects. We doctors end up causing more back pain because of our callousness by scaring the patients and inserting ideas (inception) of diseases.

In my opinion, the cause for most back pains persisting for long periods is 'iatrogenic', i.e., caused by medical examination or treatment. It's a very fancy term, but the Merriam-Webster dictionary defines it as 'induced inadvertently by a physician or surgeon or by medical treatment or diagnostic procedures'. Consultation happens to be a part of medical treatment.

Degenerative changes[4] in the spine have been found in the Neanderthal man[5] (found in 1957) and even in dinosaurs[6] (found in 1961), very similar to what we find in the human spine today[7]. The Egyptian mummies[8] have repeatedly shown to have degenerative changes. In all these periods, back pain wasn't a major contributor to disability, but today it is.

Repeatedly the clinical research studies have shown that there is very little relationship between degenerative changes of the spine and symptoms the patient feels.[9]

By definition, degenerative changes mean 'irreversible' when that is actually half the truth. Aren't we all degenerating? We should aim for slowing down that process and using the other body parts optimally to support it. Your conservative treatment, that has been dealt with in detail in this book, becomes the mainstay of your treatment.

It is you who has to address this problem. All other treatments are only supportive. Injections are worth thinking about for acute pain, so that you can lead a normal life and get on with your exercise programme. Surgery doesn't have a very definite role.

Osteoporotic Compression Fractures

As discussed elsewhere, osteoporosis is now more common than we thought before. People with osteoporosis are exposed to higher chances of getting a compression fracture. So if you are around sixty or more years of age (and post-menopausal ladies over fifty), just don't ignore it assuming it to be the normal process of ageing. It's worthwhile to rule it out. This is also common in people with cancer that has now spread to their bones. In such cases, X-ray is worth doing to rule this out.

Traumatic Fractures

These happen when there has been a trauma. If you've had a fall or any other trauma, and you have back pain, it's definitely worth getting it ruled out.

Deformity (Scoliosis)

When back pain is present with a spinal deformity like scoliosis, it may be that the curves in the spine are causing stress and pressure on the intervertebral discs, nerves, muscles, ligaments or facet joints. The back pain is not because of the bone deformity itself.

Non-prescription medicines give symptomatic relief but only temporarily. There can be a role for surgery in these cases, but it is very important to address the muscular imbalances, as that'll end up supporting the skeletal system better.

Case: Hari Gopal, seventeen years old

A seventeen-year-old boy, who had got admission to one of the top US universities, had come to me with his mother. She was very worried about how he would cope with his back. Till now, besides the deformity, his back hadn't bothered him much, but he had been advised surgery. He underwent a three-month medical strengthening and conditioning programme to address his muscle imbalances. He felt a lot more stable and stronger; and realized that the underlying back pain that he had for longer than he could remember had disappeared. He now regularly visits the university's gym to do strength-training exercises. He's changed his lifestyle, which in return has changed his life, for good.

Symptomatic Isthmic Spondylolisthesis

Spondylolisthesis is a condition in which a vertebra slides backward or forward over a vertebra below. It's usually at the base of the spine, i.e., lumbar 4, lumbar 5 or sacral 1. Spondylosis is fracture of one or both wing-shaped portions, which make the joint unstable. It can happen because of birth defect, trauma (sudden or over time), infection, disease, etc. They are divided into three grades, depending on the extent to which one vertebra slides over the other one.

It depends on how stable the affected joint is. If the joint is stable and there are no neurological symptoms like loss of strength in one or both legs, loss of bowel and bladder movements and tingling sensations in the buttock region, there is no indication for emergency surgery.

It becomes very important then to stabilize the lower back naturally by using the body more appropriately as advised in the book throughout. The focus needs to be more on stability, but the range of motion of levels not affected are equally important. There are seven vertebral spine in the neck region (cervical), twelve in the thoracic region (upper and middle back) and five in lower back region (lumbar). All these vertebrae are sitting on top of each other. Lower back vertebrae sit on stable and fused sacral vertebrae that are very stable. Vertebrae in neck, upper, middle and lower back have a certain range of movement. If any one level becomes excessively mobile or immobile, it affects the functioning of all the vertebrae above and below. That would further put more pressure and load on the affected region. If the whole spine is not addressed together, it really is not a long-term treatment. The rehabilitation exercise programme needs to be such that the whole body is addressed well.

Case: Rajni Rai (name changed), sixty-two years old

A sixty-two-year-old woman had been having generalized lower back pain for more than a decade but didn't think much of it. One day she had an episode of severe lower backache. It was bad enough to stop her from getting out of bed. The pain subsided enough in 3–4 days to let her start her daily chores again. She was advised an MRI by the doctor. The MRI showed a grade two spondylolisthesis at lumbar 4/lumbar 5 (L4/L5) region. Besides the dull lower backache, she had no other complaints. On closer look of the MRI, it showed that L4/L5 region was fused and stable. She was advised no surgery by the doctor. However, she was not given an actual plan of action to solve the problem or how to handle it.

Since the lower back pain continued, she ended up seeing me. She was advised and guided through a proactive rehabilitation programme to strengthen the lower back and also optimize the working of the rest of the spine. Over two months, she realized that the niggles in the shoulders and knees disappeared. She could now walk for more than an hour without any pain.

Spinal Stenosis

The vertebrae in the neck and the back are stacked in a manner that they form a canal within, through which the spinal cord, a continuation of brain, travels. When this canal gets compromised, the condition is called spinal stenosis. Depending on the level that the stenosis occurs in, symptoms are revealed. Spondylolisthesis (shifting of one vertebra on top of the other) would also cause spinal stenosis. The management would depend on the extent of the spinal stenosis, stability and symptoms accompanying them. As a rule of thumb, it is very important to stay active as immobility will only make the condition worse.

Non-mechanical Spine Disorders (Less Than 1 per cent)

Cancer, infection and seronegative spondyloarthritis account for less than 1 per cent of all back pains. Symptoms like weight loss should not be ignored.

Visceral Disease (1–2 per cent)

Sometimes back pain is not because of the spine at all but because of visceral diseases like infection or inflammation of the prostate, endometriosis, pelvic inflammatory disease, kidney stones, urinary tract stones, inflammation of kidneys because of infection, renal papillary necrosis, aortic aneurysm, and gastrointestinal (pancreatitis, cholecystitis and peptic ulcer disease). Other systemic diseases like Paget's disease and the parathyroid disease can also cause back pain. Good detailed history and physical examination will help the doctor pick on them. There always are accompanying symptoms as well that will point to these diagnosis. For this reason, it is advisable to always discuss the whole medical history with the doctor even though he might think it to be irrelevant to your back pain.

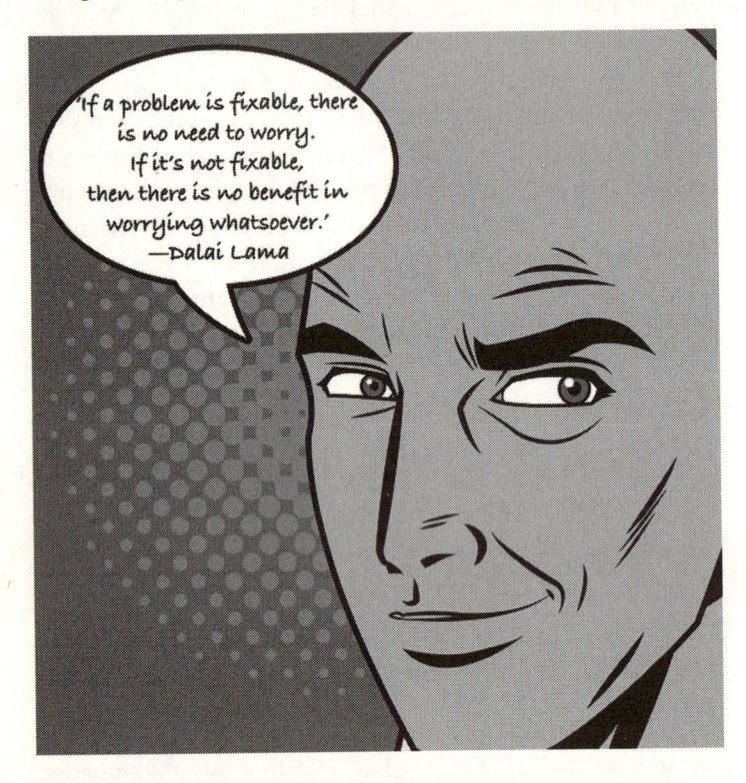

'If a problem is fixable, there is no need to worry. If it's not fixable, then there is no benefit in worrying whatsoever.'
—Dalai Lama

6

PROACTIVELY MANAGING BACK PAIN

It's not the experience that happens to you: it's what you do with the experience that happens to you.

—Aldous Huxley

Sir Edmund Hillary, after a few failed attempts at climbing Mount Everest, looking at a painting of the mountain, said, 'The more you reject me, the more determined I become. Even as Mount Everest you cannot grow any further. But I, as a human being, will continue to grow.'

'When I see it, I will believe it' is the old paradigm. Sir Edmund Hillary redefined it as, 'When you believe in it, you will see it.[1]'

GOYA (Get Off Your Arse)

In this chapter, the focus in not so much on 'why' you need to do something, but simply 'how' to do it. The 'why' has been answered throughout the book, more specifically in chapter 5. If you are in pain at this very moment, you can ignore the rest of the book and just come to this chapter and follow what is advised here.

If this book makes life more liveable for even one reader, I would consider it worthwhile.

You came into this world alone and you will depart alone. In between these two events, you experience pain in some degree or other. Some of you might have support, others might not. Some will be lucky, others won't. Don't bank on luck. If you get support, take it as a bonus. It's your pain, and you need to cater to your own needs. If you don't, no one else is going to, at least not for long. Even in the best of cases, they might feel sympathetic towards you for a while, but soon they'll be gone. You'll be left on your own to address your pain.

The sooner you acknowledge these facts, the better it will be. I prefer to talk about and focus on the reality of any given situation.

As Po's father rightly says in the film, *Kung Fu Panda*, 'There is no secret ingredient.' The same applies while addressing back pain too. I am not looking for a magical solution to your problems, because there isn't one. We will have to address multiple facets of your life to be able to treat your pain.

There are a lot of 'experts' out there, both qualified and non-qualified, who will come up with random advice. Even if there is research behind the advice doctors like me give you, it is important for you to understand that you are unique and no one knows your body better than yourself. What has worked for someone else, just might not work for you. You have been living with yourself since the time you were born. You know your body best.

What You Can Do for Yourself

There are multiple modalities that play a role in pain and all need to be addressed to relieve your back. They all interact with each other. For that reason, we won't differentiate between them. I will outline a combined plan for you. I will also talk about what not to do. It's important to remember that one set of exercises won't work for all. You will have to take a call as to what feels right. I am completely against exercise sheets given out by therapists to patients. The idea is to introduce you to some basic exercises. Based on your experience, you can continue to work with the ones that make sense to you and are acceptable to your body.

In addressing pain, a single approach won't work. It has to be a multifaceted approach to tackle it permanently or at least for a long term.

Normally, an episode of back pain is triggered because of some incident which may have happened in the past. The focus needs to be on the multiple causes that has led to the lower back becoming susceptible to pain. Most of these are lifestyle-related, that will be addressed in the latter part of this chapter.

First Aid to Relieve Pain

A majority of back pain happens because of muscle strain (spasm) and gets better in due course of time. You can make yourself more comfortable by being in a comfortable position, not fighting the posture, applying ice/heat; this will give you temporary relief.

The advice in this section is primarily for when you are in pain.

Listen to Your Body

You know your body best, better than any expert out there. You have to learn how to listen to your body. Follow the exercises mentioned here, which will make you more aware of your body. If any exercise or activity makes the pain worse, it only means you aren't ready for it yet. Stop that exercise for now, but revisit it in the next few days. Allow your pain to be your guide.

Dr George Sheehan, runner, philosopher and world-renowned cardiologist, suggested that you should 'listen to your body'. That is the trick. Some would argue that the body always wants to be lazy. That is not correct. For the first few days, it'll be a struggle to do the 'right' thing. Even if the body is in a bit of a disagreement, it'll soon settle down. The plan is to create a habit. It could take you as long as two months, and sometimes even longer, to make increased physical activity and exercises a habit, a part of your life. Till that happens, find ways where you are forced to do it. Could be peer pressure by joining groups, or a family member pestering you to exercise.

Keep Moving

Bed rest is a recommendation of the past. If there is back pain, it's important that you move, as much as your body will allow without increasing the pain. Complete bed rest is definitely not a done thing. You need to be up and about. Bed rest for more than a day or two is actually counterproductive. It not only increases pain but is also detrimental as it deactivates muscle. Muscles lose tone and become less flexible.

You might want to take time off work, but stay active. This doesn't mean you have to fight pain. It's 'active rest' that we are after. In a majority of people, back pain does not signal a serious disease or suggest that one should avoid daily activities. On the contrary, scientific studies show that healing is promoted by staying active, returning to work and exercising at an appropriate and increasing intensity.[2]

If it's too painful to move, you can start activating core muscles by doing bracing and deep-breathing exercises, which are discussed later. It's frequently noticed in chronic back pain that the sufferer has inactive gluteus maximus (buttock) muscles. They can be activated without much movement of the lower back. Gentle and slow backward and forward movements (flexion and extension) of the back, contrary to popular belief and advice, is not going to make the condition any worse.

If the affected body part and the tissue are loaded optimally, it would help in attaining correct alignment. On the other hand, if you rest a bit too long, the muscles will not adapt enough and become deconditioned. If you don't use it, you'll lose it!

On the other extreme, after a back surgery it's important to start rehabilitation at the earliest. What should stop you from working on a good posture? If you are in bed for four to six weeks, it'll only prolong your recovery as your muscles will take longer to get back to normal, if at all. If the support system around your spine isn't catered to, the results of the surgery either wouldn't be optimal or wouldn't last very long. Remember that you aren't simply a piece of furniture that a carpenter fixed. You are supposed to move. For that your muscles are very important. Get them moving.

Ice (Heat) Compression

You might have tried this earlier as well, but most people do it incorrectly. Here is the correct way:

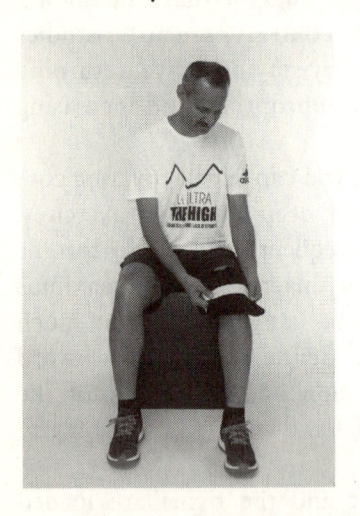

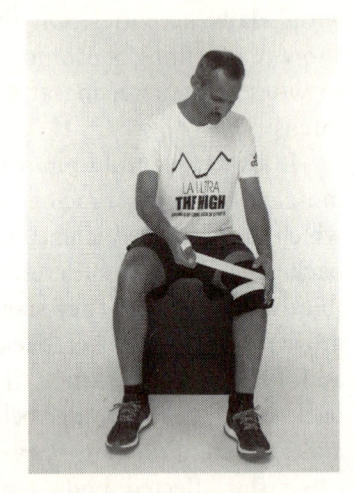

1. Get yourself two ice-gel packs, a pack of frozen peas or crushed ice in a bag. Any of these takes the shape of the body part you apply it to.
2. Place the pack on the painful area.
3. If the pain goes down the leg, it is most likely coming from the lower back or the buttock region. Apply the ice pack there.
4. Between the ice pack and your skin, place a thin layer of cloth, like a handkerchief.
5. Most people make the mistake of just leaving the ice pack on the skin. You need to compress it with a crepe bandage, towel or bedsheet. Putting ice directly on the skin can lead to a cold burn.
6. The pressure should be such that it feels firm, like a firm handshake.

7. Leave the pack for 7 to 10 minutes.
8. Remove it for another 7 to 10 minutes. Till that time, place the pack in the freezer.
9. Take out the other ice pack and repeat the earlier process three times in one sitting.
10. Repeat this three to four times a day.
11. In winter, it's better to use heat rather than ice.
12. At the end of the day, it is your choice to use ice or heat.

Lumbar Belt

Wear a lumbar support belt only for a few initial days of pain. There is no point in wearing them for longer as they provide you only with a false sense of security.[3] Lumbar belts are way too often prescribed as a quick fix for pain, but they actually give your deactivated and deconditioned muscles an excuse not to move.

Before giving you a lumbar belt to wear, it is the doctor's job to educate you on the correct usage of the equipment and dynamic posture, the amount of load that can be put on the spine while doing various activities, and the lower back muscles that need to be strengthened to avoid overloading.

Since a belt limits the angle to which you can bend on the side, these muscles become weak and taut, increasing the muscle imbalance in the lower back.[4] For this reason alone, it is a good idea to limit the usage of a lumbar belt.

Medication

You might hate taking medicines. I don't love them either, but they are there for a reason. If there is a need, they need to be consumed. We need to address pain at various points. First we need to calm it down, even if it is temporary, so that we can do things that will permanently treat it. These medicines can have side effects only if you take them over a long period of time.

OTC (over the counter) pain relievers, such as acetaminophen, ibuprofen or naproxen often work well in mild to moderate back pain. Take them for five to seven days and see how it affects the pain. Do remember, it's only masking the pain, so you do need to address other factors as well. 'A high quality review demonstrated that paracetamol was no better than placebo for lower back pain, with any perceived clinical benefit probably reflecting natural history and/or placebo.'[5]

Pain-relieving creams and sprays might be helpful in the case of muscle aches. 'Evidence shows that gels, creams and sprays are effective in providing pain relief. Gel formulations work best and they are safe alternative to oral drugs.'[6]

If you have severe pain, I would suggest you do not waste time trying to self-medicate. Seek the help of an expert. For severe pain, you might need prescription drugs.

Do remember that to get moving, you need to figure out a pain-free, or at least a reduced-pain, window. Only then will you be able to start exercising and becoming more physically active.

Gym Exercises

As much as I want you to be active, it's not a good idea to push yourself too much in the beginning. A wrong technique while exercising in the gym might bring on your back pain.

In principle, gym exercises are good, but only if they are performed under supervision, or if you know what you are doing. While you have a severe back pain, it is advisable not to do any strengthening exercises in the gym.

Again, I am a big advocate of using strengthening and conditioning exercises, but definitely not without supervision. Then there are those who believe that 'only pain kills pain'. In their opinion, you have to experience pain during exercise to get rid of pain. Please don't fall for such advice. It's simply incorrect.

Exercises in gym are covered later on in this chapter but don't rush right now. Let's first reduce the pain.

Getting Started with Exercises

The exercises and advice in this section are primarily for when you are in severe pain. All of these exercises, rather habits, should become part of your daily life as well. Continue doing these even after you are cured.

Make a Decision

1. Paste a smile on your face that stretches from ear to ear. Soon, it'll be year to year. You might start with a fake smile, but soon it will become genuine.
2. Your decision to do something about the pain is the starting point in improving the condition of your back. Since you are in control now, you'll be surprised how things turn out.
3. I need you to let go of all the thoughts brought on by reading the MRI or X-ray report or whatever your doctor said you can't do. If there is an abnormality in the MRI or X-ray that's bothering you too much, it's not the scans that we need to focus on, it's you. If the MRI or X-ray needed treatment, we could have used an eraser to do the same.
4. There are way too many pain consultants, from your guard to grandmother. Their advice might be well

intentioned, but please stop being a guinea pig for others to experiment on. Don't just try anything.
5. As much as you would want to get out of the pain at the earliest, please don't rush. You will soon see changes happening for good, but it's important to keep it slow and steady.
6. At the same time, you'll be expected to push beyond what you previously thought you were incapable of. If you remain in your comfort zone, nothing will change. Don't look for pain, but try and do just that bit more each time.
7. Stop exercising if you experience pain. There must be something wrong. Revisit that exercise at a later date. But if there is fatigue or slight discomfort, it is fine to continue.

Relax

All our pains are important. For someone it could be a pinprick and for someone else it could be an amputated arm or a severe back pain. Almost always, the extent of your pain is grossly out of proportion to how serious your problem is. It's important to stay relaxed, which is easier said than done, but if getting stressed helped, I would happily ask you to go ahead and do it. The reality is, stress only makes matters worse.

A majority of back pain happens because of muscles, tendons, ligaments and fascia that lie just under the skin. It does have a tendency to get worse if you stress. It can get better in time, but you do need to follow the tips given below.

Breathe Optimally

You can't relax if you don't breathe properly. Below is why and how.

We all take breathing for granted. Lungs are protected by the sternum (breastbone) in the front, the ribs on the sides and thoracic vertebrae at the back. They sit on a muscle called the diaphragm. A bad posture, with a slouch and rounded shoulders, limits how much your lungs can expand. When there is a muscle spasm and pain, you might hold your breath because of the subconscious apprehension of pain. It becomes a catch-22 situation. We need to break that vicious cycle at several points. Breathing normally is one of the most important ones, and the most ignored.

Also, think of your back as a building. This building, like your weak lower back, has a ground floor made of clay and, similar to your stiff upper back, has a first and second floor made of concrete. Heavy top floors put more pressure on the lower back, eventually causing it to crumble. So, the pressure on the lower back needs to be lessened.

Start with learning how to control your breath, rather than being a slave of it, as that'll help you be in better control of your pain as well. When I say 'control', I don't mean force. It's just about letting go, and allow for an easy movement out and in. When you let go, it helps you address your psychological issues as well.

Before you get on to an exercise programme, whether it is for fitness or therapeutic purposes, you need to first prioritize working on your breathing technique. This can also happen in tandem with improving your posture. Some ways in which this can be done are the following:

1. Since there could be a lot of pain when you begin, it is best not to think about the right posture while sitting, standing or lying down. Just look for a comfortable position.

2. When there is a lot of pain, there is a tendency to hold your breath, which worsens the spasms. That, in turn, increases your pain.
3. Lower back pain leads to a stiff upper back, which puts even more pressure on the lower back.
4. Try sitting on a stable chair without wheels. Close your eyes and think of letting your spine lengthen, which means letting your neck and head move away from your lower back and vice versa. This is not possible physically, but just the thought is enough. Imagine yourself to be a puppet and the string attached to the top of your head is pulling you up, while you slide forward to the edge of your chair.
5. Now take a long breath in while focusing on expanding your chest. To divert your mind from the pain, count from one to four when you breathe in.
6. Hold your breath for a couple of seconds.
7. Exhale slowly. This is accompanied by your chest coming down as well.
8. Start with this simple exercise for 1 minute every 10 minutes, but soon, you should be doing it for over 5 minutes at one go.
9. As soon as you start breathing from your chest, it'll help you relax.
10. Relief from pain might not be immediate, but it's important you keep focusing on this.

Proactive Siesta

1. Siesta[7] refers to a short nap taken in the early afternoon, often after the midday meal.
2. This exercise isn't sleeping in it's true sense. It does what sleep is meant to do. All of us sleep, but few of us

use it to recover. It is meant to unwind, release tension throughout the body and refresh the back.
3. It can be done anytime of the day.

Part 1

1. Take off your shoes and lie down on a firm surface, not one that would make you sink in, like a cushioned mattress. A yoga mat on the ground works well.
2. Lie on your back, with knees bent at a comfortable angle and your feet flat on the ground. Place your feet shoulder width apart.
3. Place your hands on your abdomen, with elbows completely relaxed.
4. Use a firm pillow or some books to support your head. The height of this headrest should be such that you feel comfortable with the thought of elongating the spine and it also doesn't tense your neck, shoulders or upper back.
5. If possible, support your neck as well. Put a rolled-up towel at the neck end of the pillow almost creating a speed breaker kind of hump. This will support the neck even better.

Part 2

1. Focus on elongating and releasing your spine, not so much straightening it.
2. Don't put any pressure. Just relax and let go. Think of your skull and tailbone moving away from each other.
3. Relax your neck. Imagine that you are losing control of your neck and let go of the tension as your skull and tailbone go their separate ways.
4. Allow your shoulders to relax.

5. Imagine your elbows moving away from the shoulders; in effect feel the lengthening of your upper arms.
6. Now let your forearms lengthen by letting your wrists go away from your elbows. Relax your wrists.
7. Now focus on your legs. Think of letting the front and back of your thighs relax, and also the calves.
8. Once you have elongated yourself, imagine your whole body floating in mid-air, rising just a few inches from the ground.
9. Let go of your feet and hands.
10. Let your feet expand by moving your toes and heel in opposite directions. Let your feet widen as well.
11. Stay in this suspended position for a count from zero to 100. Then count backwards from 100 to zero.
12. When you get to zero, get up slowly by rolling to your side.
13. Slowly you can build it up to even a count of up to 1,000 and beyond.
14. Soon this will become second nature. But keep going back to check the basics. If you keep practising it incorrectly, newer problems will creep in and there will be no opportunity to get the basics right.
15. Add optimal breathing to it once you get a hang of it.

Sit 'Easy-Peasy'

This particular exercise/posture is primarily based on the original work of F.M. Alexander (Alexander Technique), modified by Dr Wilfred Barlow, and introduced in the London College of Osteopathic Medicine by Dr John Lester. I was introduced to it in 2004 by Dr Roderic MacDonald, principal, LCOM, a gentleman who taught me an immense lot about the human body.

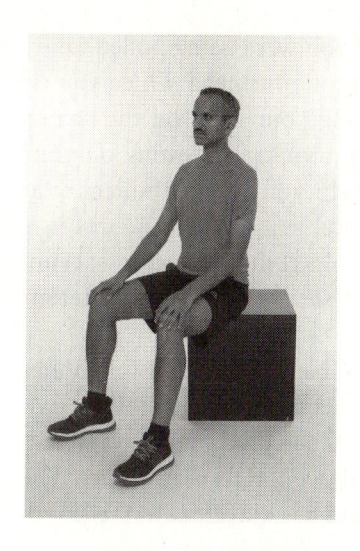

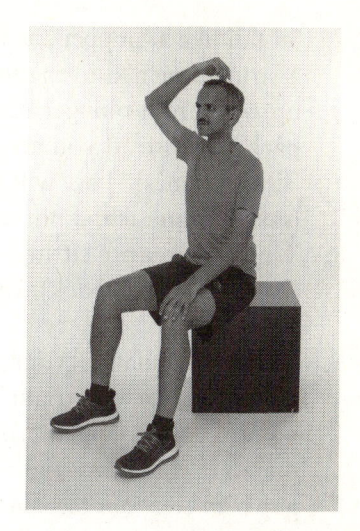

1. Sit tall on a stable surface, ideally a chair with no wheels. (I like to call 'ergonomic chairs' with wheels wheelchairs, as they are preparing you to use one permanently!)
2. There are three important 90-degree angles in your body that you need to keep a note of. The first is between your torso and thighs, the second at your knee joints and the last at your ankle joints. Have your arms by your side, hanging down.
3. Close your eyes, and remind yourself that this exercise is not about forcing anything, but about letting go.
4. Consciously relax your neck, rotate both your shoulders clockwise fifteen to twenty times and then anticlockwise the same number of times.
5. Loosen up your shoulders, with the arms dangling down. Relax your elbows.
6. Let your wrists go further towards the ground and away from your elbows.

7. Sit tall like a 'puppet', as if you were being pulled up by a string attached to the top of your head. Once you sit up, you are no longer resting your back on the chair's backrest; instead you are automatically sitting on your 'sitting bones'. This will help you become taller by at least half an inch, if not more.
8. While you are 'sitting up', think of your sacrum (base of lower back) and skull moving in different directions.
9. Form an equilateral triangle between your sitting bones (one point of the triangle) and your feet (other two points of the triangle). You'll need to spread your knees out so that they are right above the respective feet. The gap between your feet should be equivalent to the length of your thigh bone.
10. Now imagine that the puppet is not only being pulled up by a string attached on top of the head, but is being moved forward; such that it is leaning at an angle of 5 to 8 degrees. This tilt makes the centre of gravity of your body fall in the middle of the equilateral triangle being formed by your feet and sitting bones. It's almost as if you are trying to balance an upside-down cricket bat on one finger.
11. Relax your neck further and let your shoulders become even looser.

At no time does the string lose its tension. It's still pulling you up.

Nose to Knees Rocking While Sitting

This is not so much of a stretching exercise, but is good for mobility. The range is guided by pain. Do it gradually.

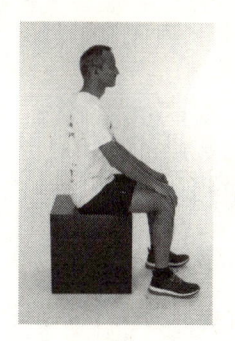

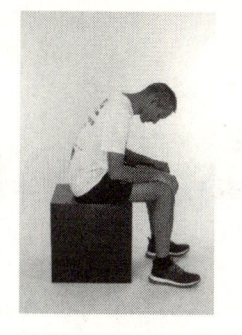

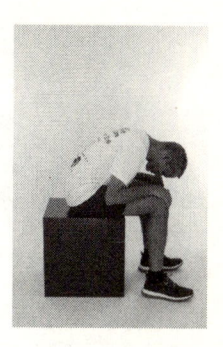

1. Sit on a stable chair (without wheels).
2. Bend forward gradually (over a count of four), bringing your nose to your knees.
3. Avoid jerky movements.
4. When you bend, think of rolling forward, one vertebra at a time.
5. Only go as far as you comfortably can. Don't push at the end.
6. Gradually (over a count of four) go back again.
7. Do this rocking movement fifteen to twenty times.
8. Again, don't hold your breath throughout this exercise. Keep your breathing normal.
9. Repeat five to six times throughout the day.
10. Do it every 30 to 60 minutes.
11. If sitting is too painful, the same exercise can be done while lying down. Bring your knees to chest and back again.
12. Important to note: Don't pull hard towards your chest.

Pelvic Tilts (Lying Down)

1. Lie on your back.
2. Bend both your knees.

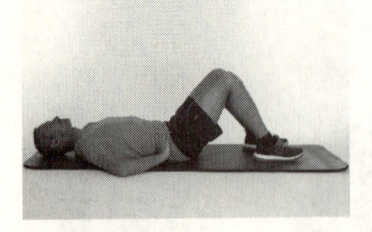

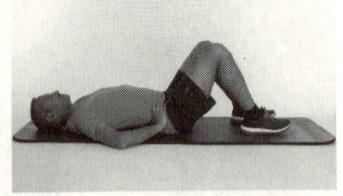

3. Put your left hand behind the small of your back and your right hand on your non-existent six-pack muscles.
4. Push your lower back against the floor. You'll notice that while doing this your pelvis rotates back.
5. Repeat four to five times throughout the day.
6. Once you get the hang of the pelvic movement, put both your hands on your pelvis (hips).
7. Now consciously rotate your pelvis backwards, which will flatten the lower back.
8. Hold for 2 seconds. Gently let go.
9. Then, consciously rotate your pelvis forwards, which will increase the arch in the lower back.
10. Hold it for 2 seconds. Gently let go.
11. Repeat it twenty to twenty-five times.

Pelvic Tilts (Standing Variation)

1. Stand up tall against a wall.
2. Have your feet shoulder width apart.
3. Keep both your hands on your waist.
4. Rotate both your hands forward and then back.
5. This time make your pelvis rotate forward along with your hands.
6. When you rotate your pelvis forward, the arch in your lower back will become even more exaggerated.

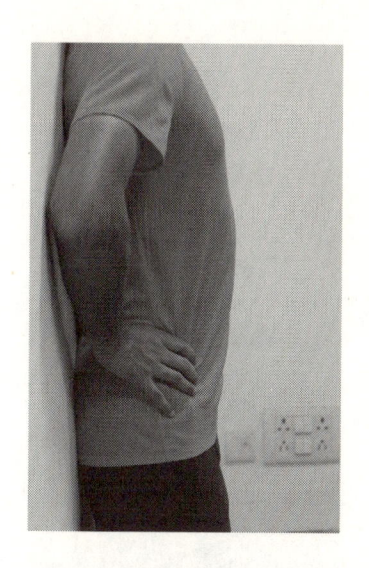

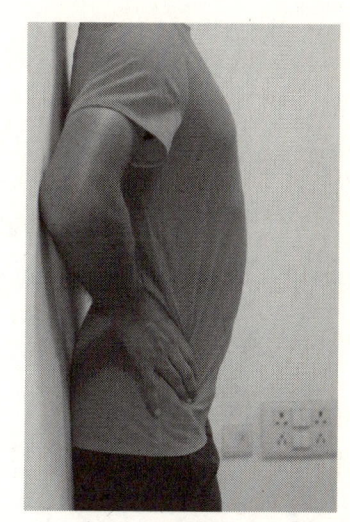

7. Now rotate your pelvis backwards.
8. When you rotate your pelvis backwards, your lower back will flatten.
9. Slowly keep rotating your pelvis forward and backward, ten to fifteen times each.
10. Do three to five sets throughout the day.

TLC (Tender Love and Care) Exercises

Anne's Alphabets

Primarily based on the original work of Anne Gibbons, my mentor in osteopathic medicine and tutor at LCOM, whom I dedicate this book to.

1. Sit tall on a stable surface, ideally a chair with no wheels.
2. Have your feet flat on the ground so that you are stable on your own feet.

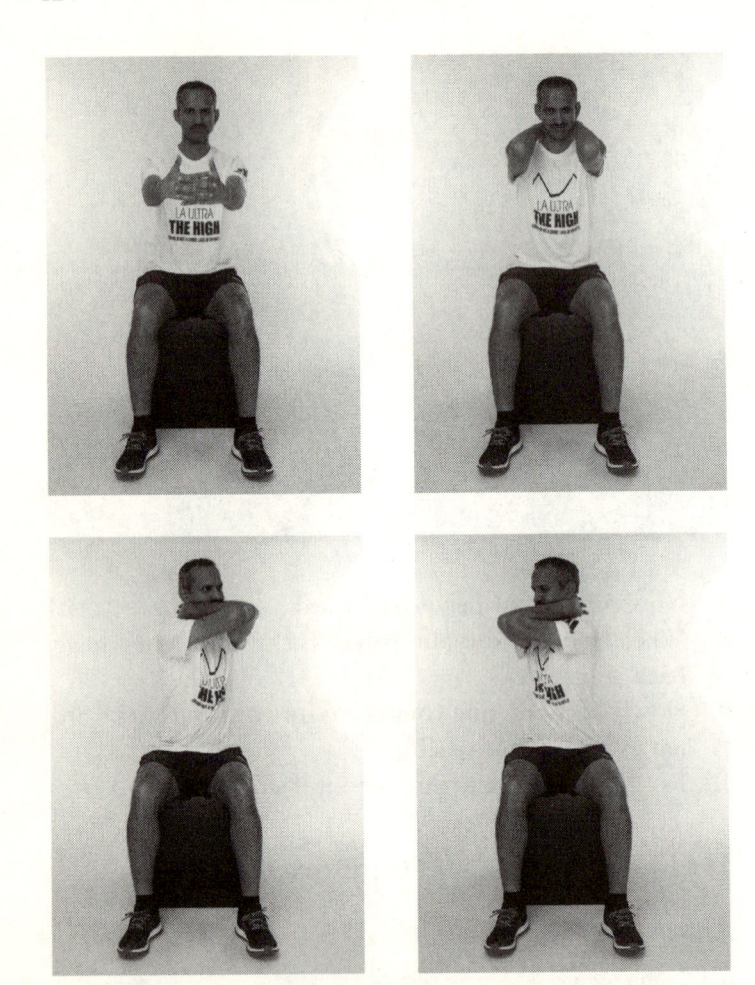

3. Interlace your fingers/hands behind your neck with the elbows pointing forward and touching if possible.
4. Imagine holding a big thick pencil between your elbows. Note, at no point should this imaginary pencil fall.
5. Now using this imaginary pencil, i.e., with the point of your elbows, slowly start air-writing lower-case

alphabets from 'a' to 'z'. They should be of font size 160 or larger.
6. It's not so much about English alphabets but about random movements that will get the upper and middle back to move, an area very difficult to mobilize.
7. Repeat this simple but important exercise every hour or two. It will help keep your upper and middle back supple.

Shoulder Retraction

1. Sit tall on a stable surface, ideally a chair with no wheels.
2. Have your feet flat on the ground.
3. Imagine a string attached to the top of your head is pulling you up.
4. Let your shoulder relax completely.
5. Raise your arms up as shown in the picture.
6. Now imagine there is an orange in between your shoulder blades and you need to squeeze it.

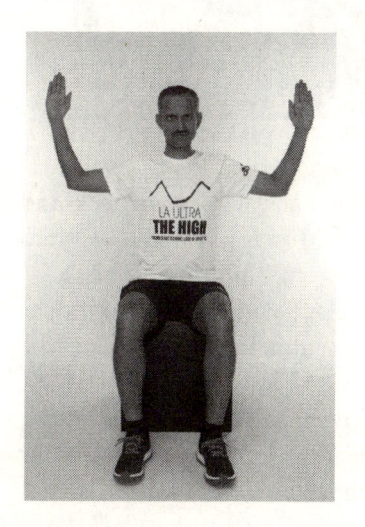

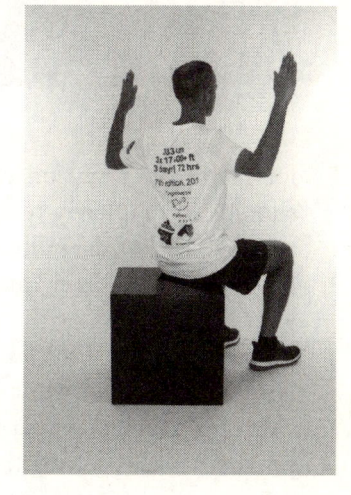

7. Hold the squeeze position for 2 to 3 seconds.
8. Relax and then repeat again.
9. It's effectively a movement of 2–3 inches.
10. Start with ten to fifteen repetitions first few times.
11. Do three to five sets throughout the day.
12. Keep increasing the repetitions over the next few days. You can soon do 100 repeats in one go.

Bracing

Primarily based on the original work of Prof. Stuart McGill, who taught me that no one posture is perfect, no two human bodies are the same and machine-based rehabilitation isn't necessarily good for the human body.

Objective: To train core muscles.

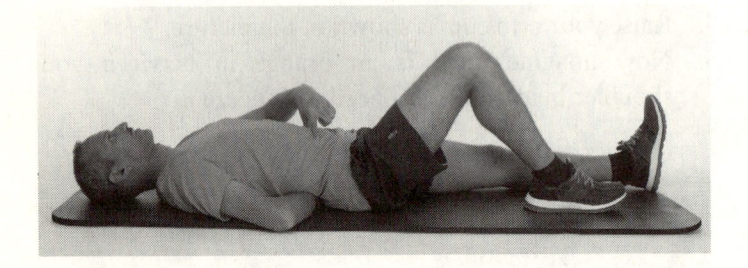

1. Lie down on a mat on your back with your neck and shoulders completely relaxed. Insert a rolled towel into the neck end of the pillowcase to support your neck.
2. Bend your right knee and place your right hand under your lower back, with the palm facing down on the floor.
3. Now try to flatten your lower back, in effect pressing your right hand underneath. You will notice your tummy muscles getting tight as well.

4. Place your index finger and the thumb of your left hand on the outer margins of the six-pack (rectus abdominis) muscles, about 2 inches away from the belly button. Imagine someone is going to punch you in your tummy. The immediate reaction is to contract your abdominal muscles. Keep them contracted.
5. Breathe through your chest by widening it and keeping your tummy tight.
6. Yes, remember to breathe. Most get too focused on just contracting the abdominal muscles.
7. Now maintain this contracted tone of the abdominal muscles without raising it up and down during breathing.
8. You will feel your whole tummy, sides and the back being worked upon.
9. Maintain this position for 7 to 10 seconds and progress gradually to hold it for longer duration.
10. Alternate with the other hand.
11. Repeat it five times throughout the day.

Note: Neither hold your breath, nor balloon your stomach out.

Butt Squeeze

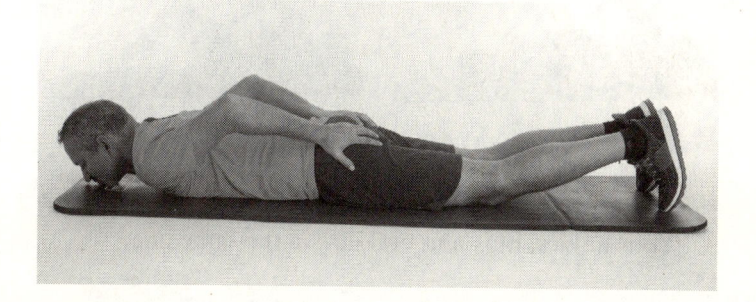

1. Lie on your stomach. If that is uncomfortable, you can do this exercise even while lying on your back, standing or sitting. This example is for lying on your stomach.
2. Imagine there is a coin between your butt cheeks and you are trying to hold it together.
3. Hold the squeeze for 10 seconds. Let go for 10 seconds and then repeat again.
4. Do this exercise ten to fifteen times at one go.
5. Repeat three to five times throughout the day.
6. Don't hold your breath while you hold the coin. Remember, it's breathing that keeps you alive, not the coin, so keep breathing.

Note: This can be done even in severe pain.

Gluteus Medius Activation

This is also primarily based on the original work of Prof. Stuart McGill.

Remember that this is not a hard-core strengthening exercise, it is only to isolate and wake up (activate) the gluteus medius muscle.

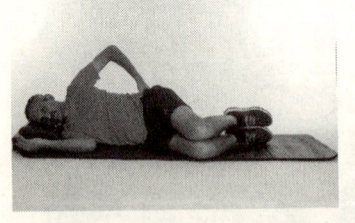

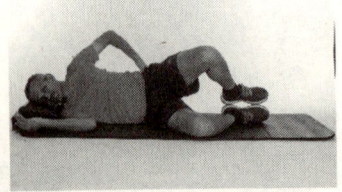

1. Lie on your right side, with your knees bent.
2. Your ankles, hips and neck are in the same line.

3. Put your thumb on the anterior superior iliac spine (ASIS). This is a projection with a pointed tip in front of your pelvis/hip bone.
4. Keeping your knees together, gradually raise your left (top) knee up only as far as the ASIS doesn't move.
5. If you are confused, just raise your knee up by 2 inches.
6. Gradually, over a count of 3 to 4 seconds, come down.
7. Repeat this fifteen times.
8. You might feel pain around the butt region.
9. Over the next few weeks, the plan is to keep increasing the repetitions.
10. In this exercise there is no need to look for a big range.
11. Do four to five sets throughout the day.

The Cat-Camel Exercise

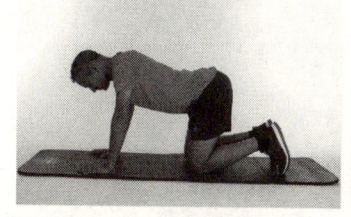

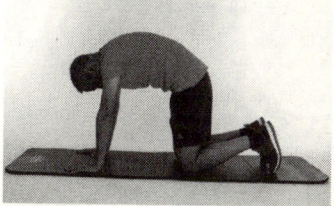

1. Get on to all fours as shown in the picture above.
2. Place your feet shoulder-width apart.
3. Your elbows should be right under your shoulders, i.e., a shoulder-width apart.
4. The gap between your knees and hands should be such that your back is parallel to the ground.
5. Now try to tilt your pelvis down slowly over a count of four, making a curve on your lower back.

6. A hollow-shaped back will form as a result of the pelvic tilt.
7. Now, tilt your pelvis the other way and round it off like a hump on your back.
8. Do this movement slowly over a count of four again.
9. Repeat this fifteen times.
10. Remember that this exercise is not intended to be a stretch, but only a mobility exercise. At the end of the ranges, don't push further.
11. Your end range is guided by your pain.
12. Do four to five sets in a day.

Flossing

This is also primarily based on the original work of Prof. Stuart McGill.

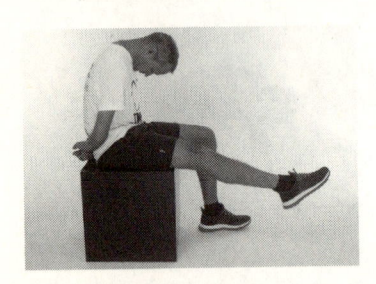

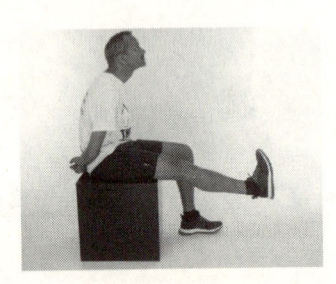

1. Think of your sciatic nerve as a string that is being pulled up and down by your head and toes. When your head is down, so are your toes. When your head is up, so are your toes.
2. Sit on a chair or a platform high enough so that your feet are flat on the ground.
3. Without bending your back, bring your chin to your chest.
4. Gradually, raise your right leg up, keeping your toes down.
5. Now bend your head down.

6. At the same time, push your toes away from you.
7. Hold that position for a second.
8. Now bring your head up and look towards the sky/ceiling.
9. Simultaneously, raise your toes.
10. If you experience pain, reduce the range. This exercise doesn't work for all. Some people with sciatica for years show improvement in days to weeks, but in some it can get worse, so just listen to your body while you do it.
11. Always remember to do this movement slowly. Never rush it.
12. Repeat it fifteen to twenty times.
13. Try doing three to five sets throughout the day.

Knee Rocking: Sideways

Note: This exercise doesn't work for all, listen to your pain, do it only if you can.

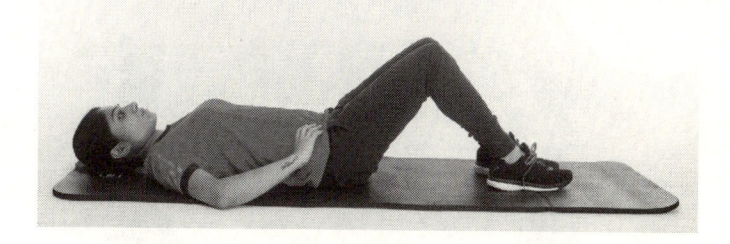

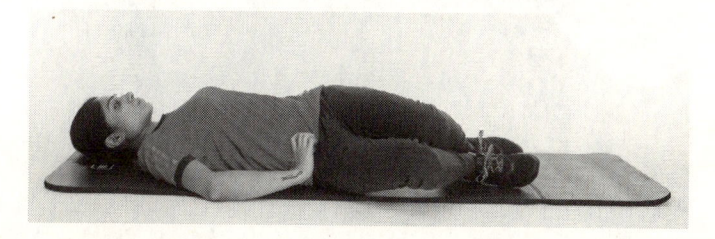

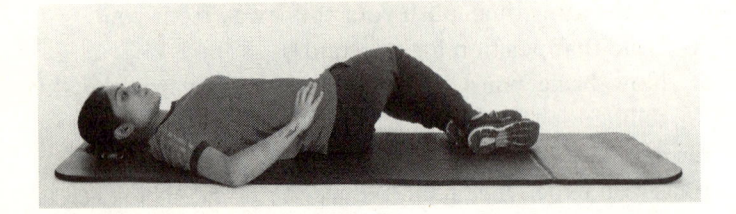

1. Lie down on your back with your knees bent at a degree that is comfortable.
2. Remind yourself about 'proactive siesta'.
3. Take your knees to one side till your butt on the other side doesn't come off the ground.
4. Now repeat the same on the other side by taking your knees to the other side.
5. Do each repetition slowly over 4 to 6 seconds.
6. At all times the range is guided by your pain.
7. Do fifteen repetitions on both sides.
8. Do three to five sets throughout the day.

Heel Raises

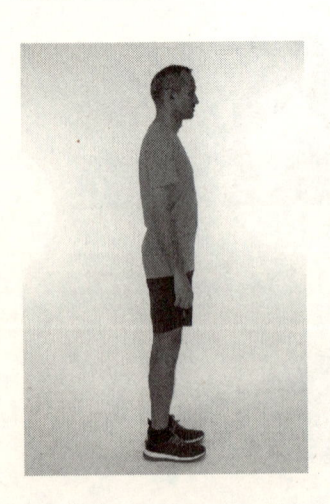

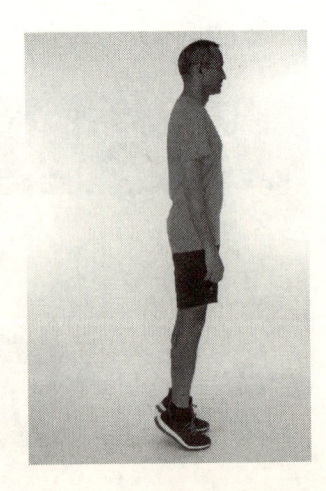

1. Stand barefoot on the floor, preferably on grass.
2. Stand tall.
3. Raise both your heels as far as you can.
4. Come down slowly.
5. Repeat ten to fifteen times.
6. Do three to four sets throughout the day.

Make Exercising a Habit

When was the last time you thought of brushing your teeth as a chore? Similarly, make these activities/exercises a part of your lifestyle. Do remember to keep the principles of 'proactive siesta', 'sit easy' and 'bracing' in mind at all times.

Brisk Walk

So, how to walk when you have back pain?

A gentle walk is a great exercise to gradually start getting your back accustomed to pressure, and to increase your confidence in yourself. Brisk walking with a focus on your swinging arms is a safe and effective exercise for back pain.[8] Interestingly enough, it is safer than a slow walk. Having said that, listen to your body, and if the pain increases during a particular pace slow down or even stop and revisit the walk the next day.

1. Go for a five to ten minute walk, depending on what feels right.
2. It's completely fine to take breaks in between.
3. Always focus on your feet and don't think too much about the distance you have completed or the speed you are going at.

4. The simple rule is, build up your distance gradually not suddenly.
5. At this point, you should walk for 30 minutes at the most.
6. Beyond that is a lot of fun, but let's not yet get all excited. We'll get back to it gradually.

Quadratus Lumborum Stretch

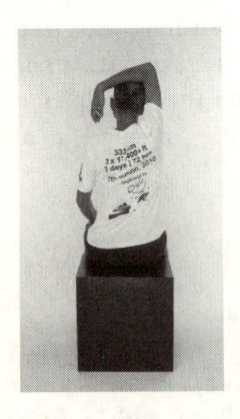

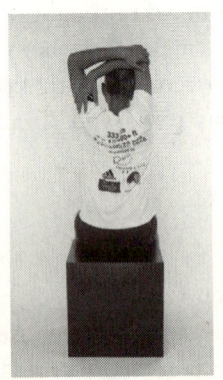

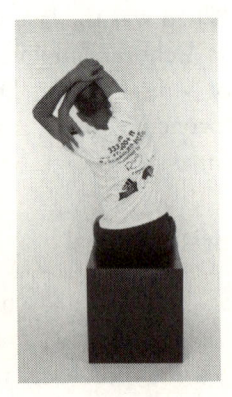

1. Sit tall with an elongated back as is shown in the picture.
2. Put your right forearm above or just behind your head.
3. Hold the right elbow with your left hand.
4. You'll already feel a stretch on the right side of the back.
5. At all times keep a straight posture.
6. Gradually start pulling your right elbow with your left hand to the left side. Go as far as comfortable.
7. Hold this position for 10 seconds.
8. Now take a deep breath in. When you exhale, you'll notice that you are able to bend further left.
9. Again hold that position for 10 seconds. Take a deep breath in and while exhaling out bend a little further.

10. Repeat three times.
11. Repeat for the other side as well.
12. Do three to five sets throughout the day.

Bridging: Gluteus Maximus Activation (Hamstring Release)

Objective: To activate the sleeping, de-activated butt muscles and release the hyperactive hamstrings (primarily based on the original work of Prof. Stuart McGill).

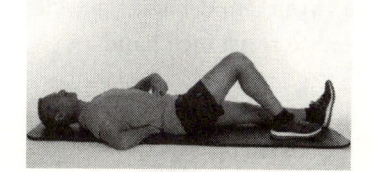

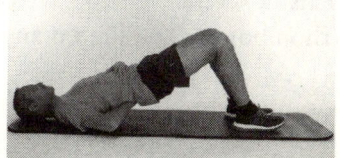

1. Lie on your back with your knee bent.
2. Your feet should be shoulder-width apart.
3. Keep your neck and shoulders relaxed.
4. Hold your brace and contract your buttock muscles as mentioned earlier even before you get started with the exercise.
5. Make sure that you use your chest to breathe.
6. Raise your buttocks up from the ground, such that your shoulders, hips and knees are in a single line.
7. Keep holding the brace and squeezing your buttock muscles.
8. You should be able to feel the muscles around the tummy.
9. Make sure that you are not straining your legs and neck.
10. Try to hold the position for 3 to 5 seconds. Make sure that you don't loosen the brace.

11. Repeat this five times. As you get comfortable with the brace, first try to increase the holding time and then the repetitions.
12. Throughout this exercise, you shouldn't hold your breath. Keep breathing normally.
13. You should consciously make an effort to release your hamstrings. It helps to have your hands over your hamstrings while releasing them.

Rowing

This exercise is to activate your mid-back muscles (rhomboids). You'll need an exercise resistance band.

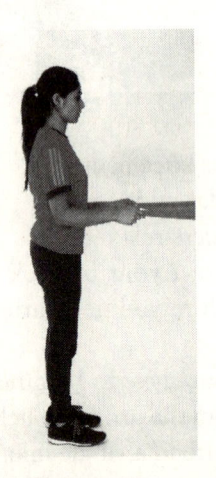

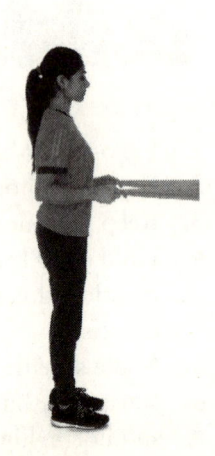

1. Loop the middle of the exercise resistance band on to a railing or door knob.
2. Sit tall on a chair (without wheels) with your feet flat on the ground (or you can stand as shown in the picture) while holding the two ends of the exercise band in both your hands.

3. Relax your neck and shoulders.
4. Remember all points from 'Sit Easy-Peasy'.
5. Gradually pull your elbows backwards keeping your shoulders and neck relaxed at all times.
6. As you pull your elbows back further, try to bring in your shoulder blades together.
7. This exercise will work the muscles in between your shoulder blades, so hold this position for 2 to 3 seconds.
8. Gradually straighten your elbows.
9. Repeat eight to ten times.
10. Do three to five sets throughout the day.

Squats

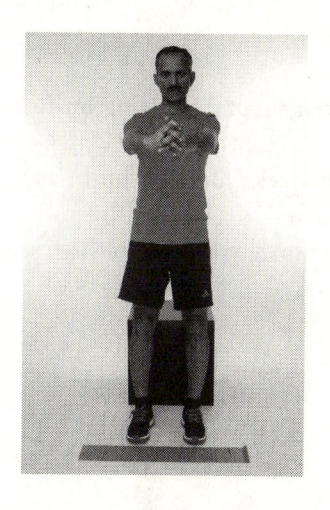

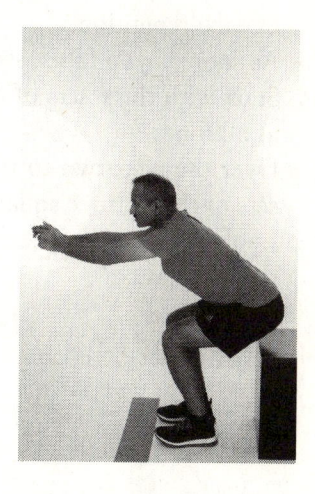

1. Stand with your toes behind a line on the floor.
2. Put a chair/stool 6–9 inches behind you.
3. Stand tall with your hands stretched out.
4. Stand with your feet shoulder-width apart.

5. Keep your feet parallel to each other.
6. Look straight ahead.
7. While squatting down, don't arch your back.
8. When you squat down, don't let your knees cross the line in front of the toes.
9. The trick is to stick your butt further back so that when you squat, your butt touches the chair/stool behind you (lower than in the photo above).
10. If you can't go all the way down till the chair yet, it's okay but fix the range of motion. It should be the same for all repetitions.
11. Squat down for 3 to 4 seconds. As soon as your butt touches the chair, come back to the original position.
12. Avoid any jerky movements and focus on the technique of each repetition.
13. As soon as you falter, stop.
14. Start with three sets of eleven squats, focusing on form at all times.
15. Over the next two to three weeks, build it up to three sets of thirty-three squats each.
16. Look at increasing the range once you can do three sets thrice a day.

Hip Adductor Stretch

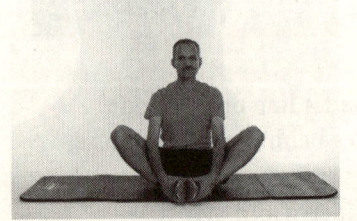

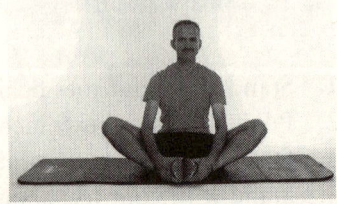

1. Sit on the floor with your legs stretched out.
2. Bend your knees and join your soles together.
3. Hold just above your ankles.
4. Place your elbows on top of the corresponding knees.
5. Push your knees down towards the floor as far as they comfortably go. Don't push too hard.
6. Keep moving your knees up and down to the maximum comfortable range. The whole range is only 2–3 inches.
7. Repeat ten to fifteen times.
8. Do four to five sets throughout the day.

Hip Adductor Squeeze

Outer thigh muscles are usually tighter and stronger than inner thigh muscles. This exercise works on your inner thigh muscles and provides stability to your pelvis.

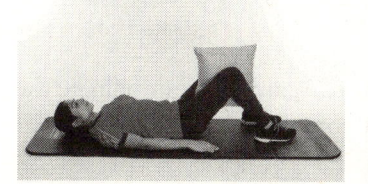

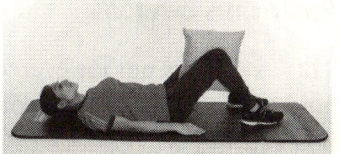

1. Lie down on your back with your knees bent and feet shoulder-width apart.
2. Place a towel roll or a ball between your knees.
3. Now squeeze the towel or ball between your knees.
4. You'll feel the inner thigh muscles working.
5. Hold it for 5 seconds.
6. Repeat twenty times each time.
7. Do it four to five times throughout the day.

Heel Drops: Calf Stretch/Activation

1. Stand tall on the edge of a raised platform, taking support of a wall or a railing.
2. Place only your toes on the platform. Rest of your foot should hang mid-air.
3. Remember this exercise is called 'heel drop', so start with that. Slowly, take your heels down as far as you comfortably can.
4. Feel the stretch in your calves.
5. Hold that stretch for 2 seconds.
6. Gradually, over a count of four, raise your heels up, so that you are now standing on your toes. Hold that position for 2 seconds.
7. Again, come down gradually over a count of four.
8. While doing this, keep your back straight.
9. Repeat this fifteen to twenty times.
10. Do three to four sets throughout the day.

Piriformis Stretch

This exercise is not for everyone. Again, let your pain be the guide. Do only as far as you comfortably can, and only if you can.

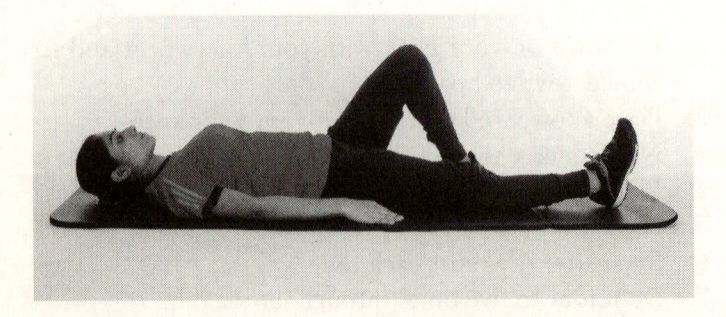

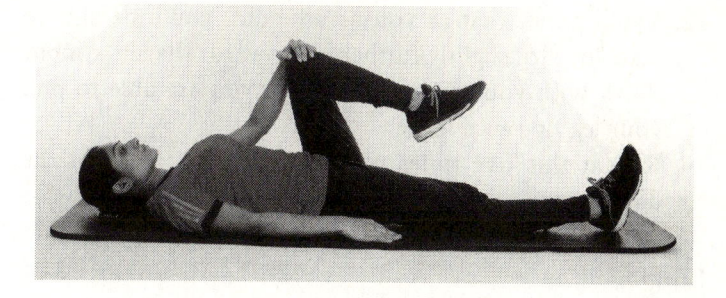

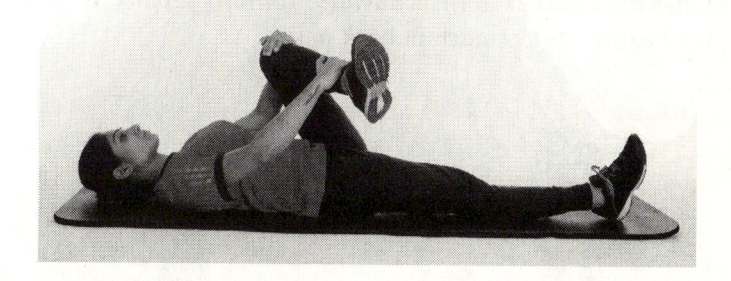

1. Lie on your back, facing up.
2. Bend your left knee.
3. Hold it with your left hand.
4. Hold the knee above your belly button.
5. Now with your right hand, hold your left leg just above the ankle.
6. Your knee stays steady above your belly button.
7. With your right hand gradually pull your left leg towards the right armpit.
8. You'll feel a stretch in your left buttock.
9. Take it only as far as is comfortable for you. Your pain should not increase.
10. While holding that stretch, take a deep breath in over 4 to 5 seconds.
11. Now slowly breathe out.

12. You'll notice that as you breathe out, you'll be able to take your leg slightly further up, towards the left armpit.
13. Work with your breathing so that you are able to pull your leg up twice more.
14. Repeat this five times with both legs throughout the day.

Lunges

Objective: This exercise is intended for hip mobility as they tend to stiffen too much in back pain.

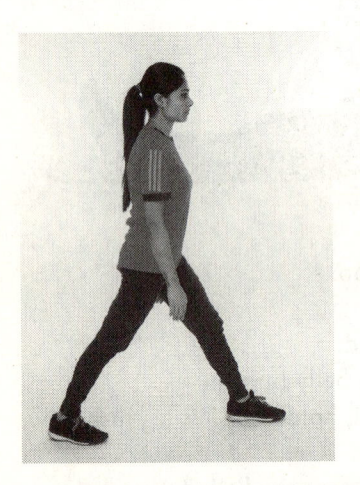

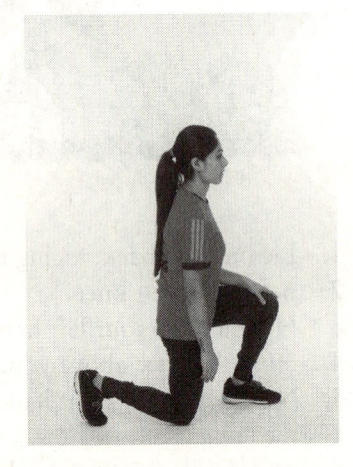

1. Keep your feet a long stride apart with the left leg in front.
2. Kneel down on your right knee.
3. Your left thigh stays parallel to the ground.
4. Keep a tall posture at all times. Keep your back straight.
5. Repeat ten to fifteen times.
6. Do three to five sets throughout the day.

Machine-based Strength Training in Gym

Machine-based exercises are good but only if you have a plan in place after a back pain episode.

Please make sure that you understand what and how to do them. It helps having the trainer or a friend supervising your technique. If the pain persists, it's a good idea to check the exercises suggested below with your doctor or physiotherapist. If you experience increased pain or sharp pain, stop immediately.

The following are the basic principles for efficient strength training:

a. Record keeping
   Always maintain a record of your strength-training sessions. For each exercise done, you need to mention machine settings, the chosen weight for the exercise and repetitions done (or time spent).

b. Duration
   A strength-training session should last 30 to 45 minutes.

c. Frequency
   Strength training three times a week is enough.

d. Recovery
   The most important time for muscles to adapt and get stronger after all that hard work is during the recovery time. Please don't do strength training exercise (especially at high intensity) on a daily basis. It will limit the muscle adaptation. Most of us take 36 to 48 hours to recover after a hard strength-training workout.

e. Body parts to exercise
   On each of the above-mentioned sessions, practise strength training for the entire body. That can be done with eight to twelve exercises.

f. Know your exercises
   You need to know which exercise works for which muscle and body part. There is a tendency to strain the whole body, especially during the last few repetitions. Relax the whole body other than the body part that's supposed to be worked in that exercise.

g. Technique
   Each repetition of any strength-training exercise should be done slowly, i.e., mindfully. Avoid any jerky movements.

h. Pacing
   Follow a 4–2–4 method. I was first introduced to it at Kieser Training. Spend 4 seconds getting the weight from starting position to end position, hold it there for 2 seconds and then bring it back to the end position over the next 4 seconds. Hold each position for 10 seconds.

i. Weight selection
   Select a weight for the given exercise. Do at least six to twelve repetitions. Don't compromise on technique of exercise to lift a heavier weight than you should.

j. Breathing
   While doing strength training, it is very important to not hold your breath. Keep your breathing easy. Inhaling or exhaling doesn't have to sync with exercise movement.

k. Intensity
   Once you are comfortable with the technique of the given exercise, you need to start increasing the intensity of the exercise. Eventually, you should be looking at exercising till local fatigue sets in and you can't carry on any more. When local fatigue sets in, either the technique or the range of motion will be compromised on.

   It's the last few repetitions, just before local fatigue sets in, that are the toughest to do, but also the most beneficial.

l. Number of sets
   One set should be enough till failure (local fatigue).

m. Sequence of exercising
   Always do strength training for your lower body first.

n. Progression
   If you can do a given exercise for 120 seconds (twelve repetitions), stop the exercise and move on to the next one after recording the time. In the next session, increase the weight by either one plate or 5 per cent, whichever is lower.

   If during the next session you are only able to do less than 60 seconds (six repetitions), stop the exercise. Next time reduce the weight by one plate or 5 per cent, whichever is lower.

Hip Abductor (Taking Thighs Away)

- Select an appropriate weight.
- Remember that this exercise is for the outer aspect of the thigh. Keep the rest of your body, especially neck,

shoulders and arms, relaxed during this exercise, throughout all the repetitions. Relax your head.
- Adjust the backrest so that you are not leaning back too much.
- Sit down, with your buttock against the backrest.
- Thigh pads should be on the outside of the thighs. Adjust them such that the lower end of the pad is above your knee joint.
- Start with your thighs together.
- Slowly, over 3 to 4 seconds, press your outer thighs against the pads and open the legs taking them apart. Avoid jerky movement.
- Take your thighs as far as possible without straining your hips and keeping your lower back in contact with the backrest.
- You'll notice that when you take your legs apart too much, there is a tendency for your back to arch forward. Don't let that happen. Your back should be in contact with the backrest at all times.
- Mark this end position as all the repetitions should be to this range.
- Hold this end position for 2 seconds.
- Slowly, over 3 to 4 seconds, take your thighs in again.
- As soon as you notice that your technique or range is faltering, stop.

Hip Adductor (Bringing Thighs Together)

- Select an appropriate weight.
- Remember that this exercise is for the inner aspect of the thigh. Keep the rest of your body, especially neck, shoulders and arms, relaxed during this exercise, throughout all the repetitions.

- Adjust the backrest so that you are not leaning.
- Sit down, with your buttock against the backrest. Thigh pads should be on the inside of the thighs. Adjust them such that the lower end of the pad is above your knee joint.
- Start with your thighs apart. Make sure not to strain them.
- You'll notice when you take your legs apart too much, there is a tendency for your back to arch forward. Don't let that happen. Your back should be in contact with the backrest at all times.
- All the repetitions should start from this position.
- Slowly, over 3 to 4 seconds, press your thighs in towards the pads and bring the legs together. Avoid jerky movements.
- Hold your thighs together for 2 seconds. This is the end position.
- Slowly, over 3 to 4 seconds, take your thighs out only to the starting position.
- As soon as you notice that your technique or range is faltering, stop.

Leg/Knee Extensions

- Select an appropriate weight.
- Remember that this exercise is for quadriceps (the upper aspect of the thigh). Keep the rest of your body, especially neck, shoulders and arms, relaxed during this exercise, throughout all the repetitions.
- Backrest should be adjusted such that the centre of your knees are in line with the pivot of the machine. You might have to go in and out of the machine and readjust a few times to get this right.

- Sit down, with your buttock against the backrest. Your knees should be shoulder-width apart and both legs parallel to each other.
- Starting position should be at a 90-degree angle at the knee joints.
- Slowly straighten your legs. Avoid jerky movements.
- Hold this end position for 2 seconds. Avoid locking the knees in this end position.
- There is a tendency to arch your lower back when the weight is too much or you are tired. Please avoid doing that.
- Maintain the same gap between the knees throughout all the repetitions. Keeping a small soft ball or a pillow could help.
- Again, slowly lower your legs.
- At the end, avoid letting the weights to touch down.
- As soon as you notice that your technique or range is faltering, stop.

Seated Leg/Knee Curls

- Select an appropriate weight.
- Remember that this exercise is for the hamstrings. Keep the rest of your body, especially neck, shoulders and arms, relaxed during this exercise, throughout all the repetitions.
- Backrest should be adjusted such that the centre of your knees are in line with the pivot of the machine. You might have to go in and out of the machine and readjust a few times to get this right.
- Your knees should be shoulder-width apart and both legs parallel to each other.
- Sit down, with your buttock against the backrest. The starting position should be with the knees fully

straightened. Please avoid arching your lower back. Keep it flat against the backrest.
- Slowly, over 3 to 4 seconds, bend your knees to a 90-degree angle. Avoid jerky movements.
- Hold this end position for 2 seconds. Avoid bending your knees beyond 90 degrees.
- Again, straighten your legs.
- There is a tendency to arch your lower back when the weight is too much or you are tired. Please avoid doing that.
- Maintain the same gap between the knees throughout all the repetitions. Keeping a small soft ball or a pillow could help.
- At the end, don't let the weights to touch down.
- As soon as you notice that your technique or range is faltering, stop.

Prone Leg Curl

- Select an appropriate weight.
- Lie down on your tummy, with your face down.
- Your knees need to be in line with the pivot of the machine.
- The weight pad should be in contact with your calves.
- Slowly, over 3 to 4 seconds, bend your knees, raise your heels towards your buttocks.
- Raise your calves but don't arch your back. Stop if this happens.
- Hold this end position for 2 seconds.
- Slowly lower your legs to the starting position.
- Start the next repetition without letting the weights to touch down.
- As soon as you notice that your technique or range is faltering, stop.

Leg Press

- There are two kinds of machines for this exercise. In some, the footplate component of the machine moves and the back stays stationary, whereas in others, the back component moves and the footplate stays stationary. It's important that you make yourself aware of it before you start.
- Select an appropriate weight.
- Adjust the machine's position. Make sure you don't strain your lower back while doing this exercise. Adjust accordingly.
- Sit down, with your buttock against the backrest.
- Now place your feet on the footplate keeping both your feet parallel to each other, with a shoulder-width gap in between them.
- At times, it helps to have a pillow in between your knees as there is a tendency to take the knees out when doing the exercise. Keep them shoulder-width apart.
- Slowly extend your legs, stopping just short of locking your knees at the end when they straighten.
- Hold this end position for 2 seconds.
- Slowly return to the starting position, making sure that you don't let the weights touch down.
- As soon as you notice that your technique or range is faltering, stop.

Seated Chest Press

- Select a weight that is easy for you to start with. First get your technique right before adding more weights.
- Remember that this exercise is for the chest. Keep the rest of your body, especially neck, shoulders and

arms, relaxed during this exercise, throughout all the repetitions.
- Adjust the seat height and backrest such that when you hold the bars, your shoulders don't shrug. Your wrists should be at shoulder level, not above or below.
- Sit down, with your buttock against the backrest.
- There is a tendency to arch your lower back when the exercise becomes difficult. Please avoid that.
- Also avoid shrugging your shoulders. Relax them.
- Slowly push your hands forward. Even if the machine is designed to only move forward, make a mental note to bring your wrists together at the end.
- Hold the end position for 2 seconds.
- Slowly come back to the starting position, making sure that you don't let the weights touch down.
- As soon as you notice that your technique or range is faltering, stop.

Upper Back 1: Rowing

- Select a weight that is easy for you to start with. First get your technique right before adding more weights.
- Sit down erect, leaning slightly forward like a puppet.
- Hold the handle grips. Keep your elbows shoulder-width apart and forearms parallel to each other.
- There is a tendency to arch your lower back when the exercise become difficult. Please avoid that.
- Imagine that there is an orange between your shoulder blades that needs to be squeezed. Throughout the exercise focus on squeezing this orange.
- Also avoid shrugging your shoulders. Relax them.
- Hold the position for 2 seconds.

- Make sure not to raise your elbows.
- Slowly go back to the start position, making sure that you don't let the weights touch down.
- Make sure that throughout the exercise you keep a straight posture and don't arch your lower back.
- As soon as you notice that your technique or range is faltering, stop.

Upper Back 2: Pull Down

- Select an appropriate weight.
- Hold the handle grips and sit down.
- Sit down erect, leaning forward slightly like a puppet.
- Slowly pull your elbows and wrists down.
- Imagine that there is an orange between your shoulder blades that needs to be squeezed. Throughout the exercise focus on squeezing this orange.
- Avoid shrugging your shoulders. Keep them in a neutral position at all times.
- Hold the position for 2 seconds.
- Let go slowly, making sure that you don't let the weights touch down.
- Keep sitting straight, without getting up, during every repetition.
- Make sure that throughout the exercise you keep a straight posture and don't arch your lower back.
- As soon as you notice that your technique or range is faltering, stop.

Back Extension

- Select an appropriate weight.
- While sitting, take your buttocks all the way back.

- Bend a little forward while sitting. This is the starting position. Slowly push the weight back only using your lower back.
- Hold the end position for 2 seconds.
- Slowly come back to the starting position. Make sure that you don't let the weights touch down.
- As soon as you notice that your technique or range is faltering, stop.

Abdominal Crunch

- I strongly recommend not to use the abdominal crunch machine as most cause back pain while doing this exercise rather than prevent or rehabilitate it.
- Crunches/sit-ups in any case are not recommended.

Exercises for Back Pain During Pregnancy

During pregnancy, because of physical and hormonal changes, a poor posture becomes second nature, especially if strengthening isn't done. Posture will only improve if muscles can hold the body up.

All the exercises mentioned above are useful and safe but please make sure to get professional supervision to understand them properly and then focus on the technique.

Exercises Specific to Pregnancy

All exercises mentioned above are useful in pregnancy too.

Kegel Exercise

This exercise targets your pelvic floor muscles which supports the bladder, uterus and bowel. This exercise reduces the chances of having urinary incontinence (loss of bladder control). Moreover, pelvic floor, being an integral part of your core muscles, helps in strengthening the lower back region as well.

1. Sit straight on a stable chair (without wheels).
2. Imagine that you have to pass urine, but you are stopping it by contracting the muscles in the pelvic and vaginal region.
3. Hold for a slow count of five and then relax.
4. Breathe out as you release the muscles.
5. Repeat this ten to fifteen times.
6. Do three to four sets throughout the day.

Exercising in Pain

The commonest practice in pain is for the therapist or doctor to share a sheet of recommended exercises. Mostly, the same set of exercises is handed to all. I also have mentioned exercises earlier in this chapter, but you need to be smart in picking out the ones that work for you. Listen to your body and pain, and see what is the best option for you.

Even if it's specific, not enough attention is paid to technique. If the correct exercise is done incorrectly, it can do more harm than good. This makes the sufferer lose confidence in the exercise. They start accepting their fate, i.e., they simply are meant to suffer now. So you can see how the physical and psychological are related.

Unlike what my 'expert' doctor colleagues want you to believe, you know your body best. Only you know how bad the pain is. It's your call on how much to push, once you have been empowered through more knowledge. If some pain comes along, after some awareness, you'll know how much is good for you and what could be harmful. Again, this only sets in once you have been given that confidence and explained about the body.

Another point to be kept in mind is that each day your body will respond differently to exercise. The first few times it might revolt and cause more pain. Do not worry. Your condition won't get worse if you keep your movements slow and easy. It's similar to when someone goes for a 5-km walk first time ever. Everything just hurts. Your system has undergone shock by the sudden change of level of physical activity. Once the body calms down, it starts feeling a lot easier. It is very understandable, but please don't panic. You need to be patient with this approach as there is no magic pill, nor is there any short cut.

Exercises to Improve Posture

Most of us want to improve our bad postures by exercising. Practice can make a man perfect at imperfection. It actually ingrains the wrong techniques and makes the posture even worse. You start doing any activity in the same pattern that has now become a habit for you. That needs to be addressed. You will not know unless there is awareness about the same.

It's not about what you do; it's also about how you do it.

There is first a need to correct the imperfection by doing exercises under correct supervision, with correct techniques and posture. Once you've gone through this book, I would trust you with the job a lot more than the trainers. It's not rocket science. It has to work, and it will work.

The very first workout for all of us was when we came into this world and took our first breath. If, for some reason, we didn't breathe the nurse slapped us on our backs and we screamed. A large percentage of us wouldn't have made it out of the labour room if it wasn't for that slap. It helped us then to not only have good supervision, but an intervention. The same is needed today.

I like to use the example of running. If you pick up running to get fit, pretty soon you'll get hurt because you were not fit enough to run in the first place. You would have run at a younger age, say when you were three. It's difficult now as your neck is tense and pointing forward, your shoulders are rounded, your chest is caving in and your feet stick out like Charlie Chaplin's. Running might not end up hurting the body parts directly involved in posture, but other parts that compensate. Lower back pain or knee pain could come visiting. Before you start running to get fit, it is imperative to first become fit to run. Otherwise injuries are bound to happen.

It is advised that before you run, start walking. It is a great exercise for back pain. It's easier to think about posture while running. Once your posture improves while running, naturally your posture while running will become a lot better.

Gravity happens to be that resistance against which we need to work. As infants, and later as kids, lifting our head or sitting up came naturally to us. We simply let our bodies relax and let go, rather than forcing against gravity by tensing up. The movement happened smoothly.

We need to get back what we were born with. It's easier than it's made out to be. We've worked hard to get into this mess. It will take time, you just need to persevere.

Proactively Managing Back Pain

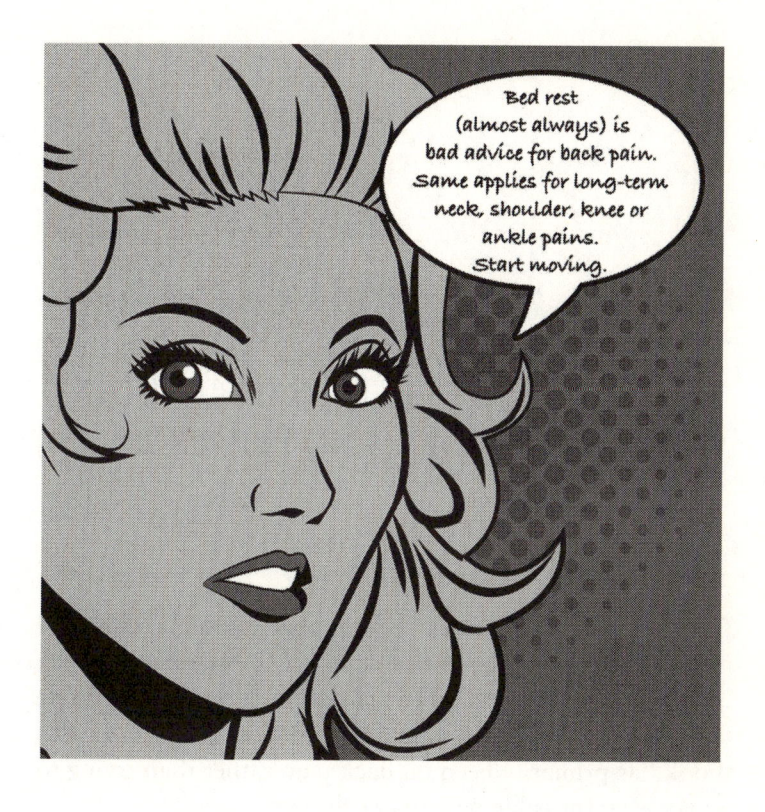

7

THE THREE MUSKETEERS: FOOT (AND ANKLE), KNEE AND HIP (FKH)[1]

Low back pain causes more global disability than any other medical condition known to mankind.[2] Neck pain is ranked fourth.[3] That is reason enough to dedicate an entire book to back pain alone. Hence, the focus of this book has primarily been on back pain rather than trying to cover every possible pain under the sun.

Knee and hip pains aren't very far off from the top spot. Together, they are the eleventh highest contributors to global disability.[4] Hence, this chapter is dedicated to foot (and ankle), knee and hip pain.

The spine is the chassis of the human body. The rest of the body is built upon it. Your legs are like the wheels of your very complex machinery. There is no point in discussing the skeletal structure of the legs, without understanding their functionality.

In order to move from A to B, whether it is walking, running, cycling or even swimming, the feet (and ankles), knees and hips need to work in synchronization. I like to call this combination of 'foot-knee-hip' (FKH) the 'Three Musketeers'.

If you visualize a human wooden puppet with joints at the feet (and ankles), the knees and the hips, you'll notice that when you make this puppet walk, all these three joints move together in sync. If any one joint doesn't move well, the pressure will fall on the other two joints. Soon enough, one or both of remaining joints will give way under the pressure, or it may also impact the structure of the puppet elsewhere on the body.

The same principle applies to us. We need to get our feet and ankles moving. Remember, the skeleton is a stationary structure. None of the bones move in isolation. They are held together by ligaments. The muscles and tendons, with a lot of help from the ligaments, help move the skeleton. The message to move comes via the nerves, only after an initial spark from the brain.

The Forgotten Feet (and Feat)

Our lifestyle today is more or less sedentary. We take our feet and ankles for granted. It may surprise you to know that each foot and ankle consist of twenty-six bones, fifty-seven joints, thirty-two muscles, and a network of ligaments. That's about a quarter of the quantity in the entire human body. (For ease of use, we will use the term foot instead of foot and ankle).

This is reason enough for us to take good care of our feet but sadly we tend to neglect them.

One could perhaps argue that one has been walking since childhood and surely has perfected the art by now. How dare then do I have the audacity to tell you that you have not been moving your feet properly? Let me push my luck. Would you believe me if I told you that you don't even *know* how to walk? Most of you simply shuffle!

Here is a challenge for you to demonstrate that you haven't been using your feet well enough. Let's do some simple heel raises.

Self-assessment:

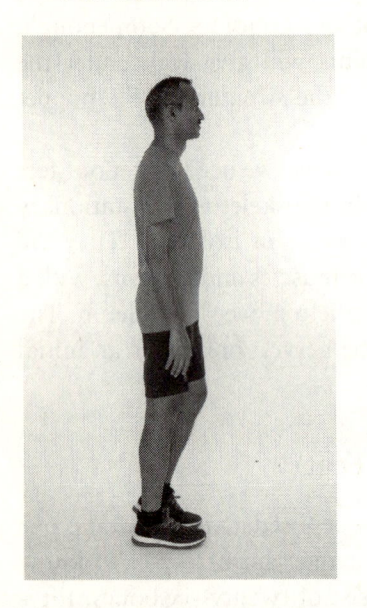

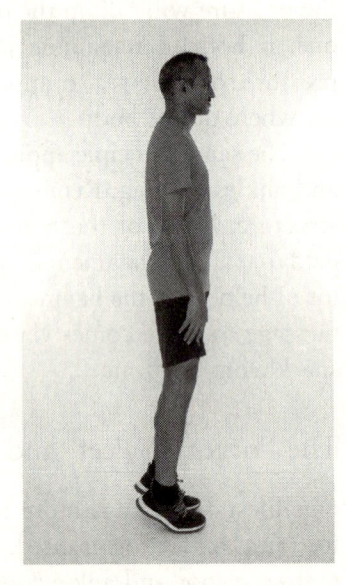

a. Take the support of a wall, a table or a chair.
b. Raise your left leg off the ground.
c. Now keeping your right knee straight, slowly come up all the way on the toes of your right foot.
d. Hold for a second or two.
e. Slowly come down again.
f. Repeat twenty to fifty times.
g. Now repeat with the left leg.
h. Do four sets of fifty with both legs.

Movement advocates recommend that you should walk 10,000 steps a day. In that case, the 400 heel raises would be equal to a brisk walk in the park. Did you find this rather simple movement awkward to do? Did you feel the burning sensation in the calf like you have never felt before? Was it easier to do on one leg compared to the other? If you have answered 'yes' to any of these questions, it demonstrates that besides not moving your feet enough, you are lop-sided too. Your calves and small muscles of the feet get fatigued easily doing this basic activity.

What limits our foot (and ankle) movements are tight calf muscles and vice versa. There are two sets of calf muscles, one (gastrocnemius) starts from above the knee and the other (soleus) starts from just below the knee joint. Together they form the calf, which further forms the Achilles tendon, which is attached to the heel bone.

Tight calves restrict the movement of the feet. This leads to a domino effect which leads to an injury starting anywhere from the feet, the knees, the hips, lower back or the upper back.

In a situation like this, the range of motion of the knee will neither be full nor fluid. This will put pressure on the knees when you stand, walk or run. This will further lead to excessive straining of your hamstrings and hip flexor muscles, making it subconsciously uncomfortable for you to stand upright. Both hamstrings and hip flexors have been shortened because of long sitting hours.

The combination of these factors puts even more pressure on your hips and lower back. You'll often catch yourself standing in a position with your knees and hips locked, which I like to refer to as a 'lazy position' because you tend to switch off your muscles. Soon enough, it becomes a habit and your muscles can't do much even if you want them to. If and when they do, there is such an immense amount of muscle imbalance that over time it only leads to injuries. That's exactly what happens when you suddenly have the urge to be fit after being a slob for decades.

The Charlie Chaplin Stance

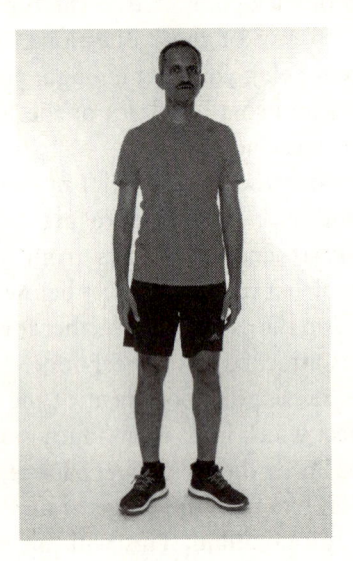

Long periods of sitting over decades makes you stand like Charlie Chaplin. Don't be offended by my remark. Instead, take umbrage at the state you have put your body into.

Self-assessment:

a. Stand up right now. Yes, now. See for yourself.
b. Walk in the same spot for 10 seconds or so.
c. Now check how your feet are placed? Are your toes pointing outwards like my favourite actor Charlie Chaplin?
d. Hence the Charlie Chaplin stance.

Now sit down comfortably. You'll notice that most probably you'll have one of the two postures. Either you'll cross one leg over the other or you'll have your legs wide apart. In both cases, you are putting pressure on the outside of your thighs (outside muscles of the quadriceps). If you happen to have one leg over the other, simply uncross and you'll notice that it's very difficult for you to sit with your legs close to each other. So when you now stand, you'll maintain the same position as you have while sitting down. Basically, by practising this for decades, you have perfected the art of imperfection.

Overpronation and Flat Feet

In addition to this, we humans have arches on the inside of the feet because of our ancestors' fascination with climbing trees. Since most of us aren't climbing trees any more, our foot arches have become weaker. When we stand, these arches collapse.

You would have often heard people self-diagnose themselves with flat feet. This isn't really a diagnosis because flat feet themselves aren't too much of an issue. Overpronation is.

Overpronation is an extensively used term today and again thought of as a diagnosis. Let's first understand what pronation means. While walking or running, pronation happens when we land on the heel of the foot first and then transfer our body weight to the forefoot, and the foot naturally rolls inwards. Rolling in to an extent is normal, which is called neutral, and a high percentage of people pronate to a 'normal' extent. However, in many cases, feet roll in excessively, which then is termed as over-pronation.

Self-assessment:

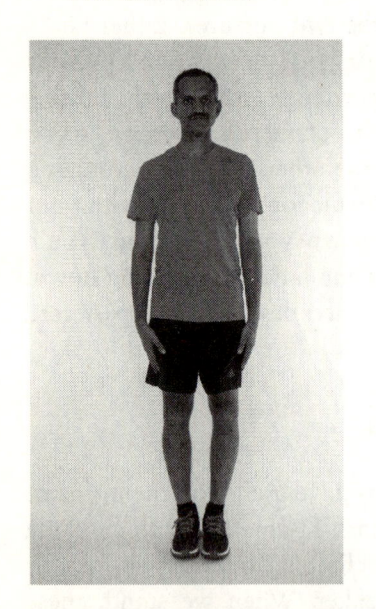

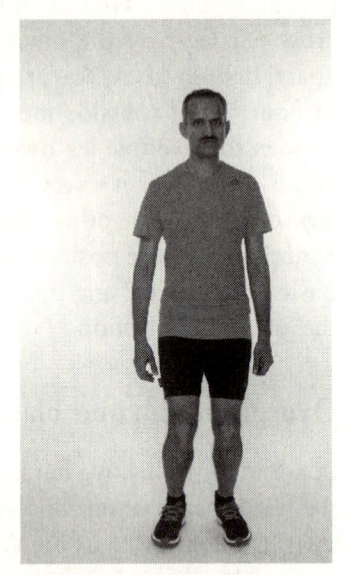

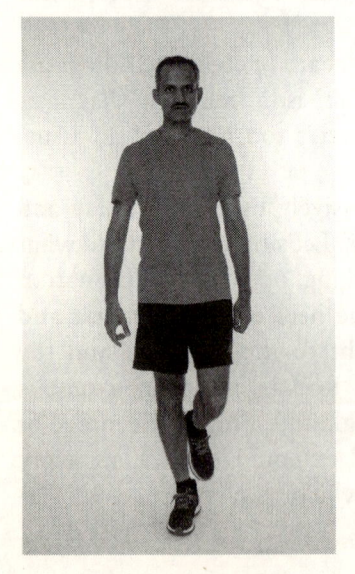

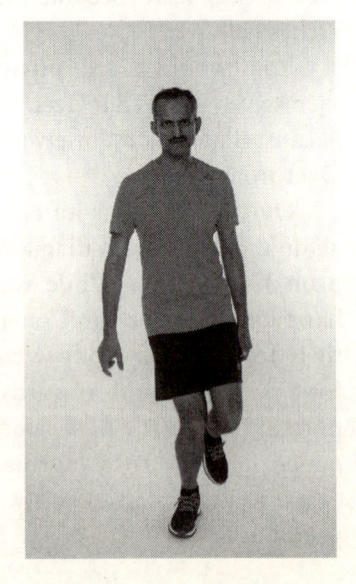

a. Stand in front of a mirror wearing shorts that don't cover your knees.
b. Squat down some five–ten times.
c. Then look in the mirror at the inside arches of the feet.
d. Do the arches collapse when you squat down?
e. If yes, look at your knees in the mirror during the next squat. They will tend to roll in as well.
f. Now come up and squat on one leg since you walk or run with one leg at a time.
g. Now look at the inside of the arch of the foot planted flat on the ground. Does it collapse?
h. If yes, does the knee roll in and look unstable when you squat?
i. You might also see that your hip of the same side also tends to drop down a bit.

Flat foot is static, i.e., when you are stationary while standing up; but overpronation is dynamic, i.e., while walking or running. It is incorrect to use these terms interchangeably. People with flat feet can have a neutral running style.

The weakening of the small muscles in the feet and the bigger muscles of the legs and buttocks leads to both flat feet and overpronation. Strengthening them is the long-term solution. The short-term solution is to have shoes that cater to this shortfall.

In overpronation, the foot—having landed on the heel—starts to roll in and by the time the whole weight is shifted to the front of the foot, the foot has rolled in even further. The arch of the foot could have collapsed to varying degrees by now. In overpronation, the knee tends to roll in as well, which further leads to the hips and the lower back rotating inwards with each step taken.

If you happen to have a Charlie Chaplin posture, besides the alignment being thrown off, the amount of range that has to be travelled by the foot while bearing the full weight on the forefoot is compounded. In combination, overpronation and the Charlie Chaplin stance are a perfect recipe for disaster and this also affects the lower back.

Toe Curls

It is the simple things in life that are most meaningful. Here is a simple drill that will help you wake up the small muscles of your feet that you had forgotten about and get your foot arches back in shape again.

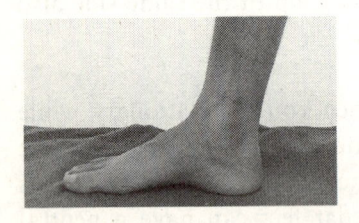

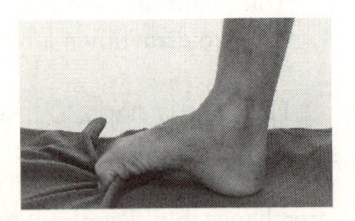

a. Stand barefoot on a piece of cloth.
b. Focus on one leg at a time.
c. Curl your toes up so that you hold the cloth between your toes and raise it off the ground.
d. Hold it for 2 to 3 seconds and then let go.
e. Repeat twenty times.
f. Repeat with the other leg now.
g. Do five sets throughout the day.

You may find that your foot cramps up. This is simply because the muscles haven't been used in a long time. Start with fewer repetitions and gradually build them up. You'll be surprised that in about a month, your foot arches will be a lot more responsive to your movements such as walking, running, etc.

The Role of Appropriate Footwear

There are two ways to improve your overpronation and flat foot, whether it is natural or artificially created by poor posture. The question here is not that which one is better than the other. Both need to be dealt simultaneously to cater to long-term and short-term effects. One approach will be able to make a bigger difference in tandem with the other, rather than working solo.

The natural way is to get the muscles to start working the way they should. For that, various drills and exercises are suggested in this book, focusing on your foot arches, calves, quadriceps, hamstrings, ilio-psoas muscle, ilio-tibial band and the lower back.

You spend a quarter to half of your life in shoes. In almost all cases that's even more than the time spent in your bed. The importance of appropriate footwear, therefore, is paramount. It becomes imperative to support your efforts with exercises even when you are not thinking about all those muscles.

If the inside of your shoes isn't providing enough support to the feet and lets them roll in (over-pronate) with each step, this contributes to your foot, knee, hip and back pain. If that is not happening already, it soon will. This is relevant for work and casual shoes even more than sports shoes, as you might wear those only while going for a run or to the gym.

Self-assessment for proper shoes:

a. Stand barefoot in front of the mirror.

b. If your arches are rolling, followed by your knees, you need shoes that support your foot arches.
c. Find a shoe that you think supports the inside of the foot.
d. Squat again wearing those shoes and see how much your feet roll in.
e. If the rolling has reduced markedly, there's your shoe.
f. Do try several others from different brands till you find the right fit.

The shoe needs to feel right to you as well. At the end of the day, my role is that of a matchmaker. I am simply trying to match your feet to the kind of shoe that will be an ideal partner. You then need to go on a date with the shoe to see if it actually works for you.

Rest of the Foot and Ankle Anatomy and Other Common Injuries

The ligaments on the outer and the inner portion of the ankle play a very important role in stabilizing the ankle joint and the rest of the body while standing, walking, running, dancing or jumping on them.

Lateral Ligaments of the Ankle

The outer aspect of the ankle joint comprise three ligaments, the relatively weaker anterior talo-fibular ligament (ATFL), the stronger posterior talo-fibular ligament (PTFL), and the calcaneo-fibular ligament (CFL).

These ligaments suffer the maximum number of injuries during sporting activities.[5] This kind of injury primarily happens with an outstretched, rolled-out foot. The imbalance between the muscles also contributes to the chances of getting this injury. Wearing wrong or inappropriate shoes adds to the problem.

Medial Ligaments of the Ankle

Ligaments on the inner aspect of the ankle joint (deltoid ligaments) consist of three superficial and two deep components, fanning out in a triangular fashion. This provides significant support to the inner side of the ankle and also supports the arch in the inner side of the foot.

In either of the cases, X-rays should be requested if a fracture is suspected. A radiologist, who is adept at investigative ultrasound, is highly recommended.

Plantar Fasciitis

Plantar fasciitis is the commonest cause for heel pain. Most people associate a heel spur (a bony prominence that can sometimes be seen on an X-ray) with heel pain, but there seems to be almost no correlation. Remember that bones are living tissues. They keep moulding themselves based on the pressures that they are put under.

The Achilles tendon is a continuation of the calf muscles that finally attaches to the heel. Plantar fascia is the flat band of tissue that connects your heel bone to your toes. Both calf muscles and plantar fascia, when they become tight, almost get into a tug of war. This 'rope' is attached right in the centre, i.e., at the heel. When both calf and plantar fascia tug hard, the pressure falls on the heel. This is why the heel, or the bottom of your foot, hurts when you walk or remain standing.

Overpronation, high arches or flat foot, long walking, standing or running on hard surfaces and/or wearing inappropriate shoes, adds to the problem. A conservative approach addressing all of the above, along with correcting muscle imbalance, works really well. Injections or surgeries are very rarely needed.

Rest of the Knee Anatomy

The knee joint, unlike the hip joint, is not a ball-in-a-socket joint. It's not stable by design. One bone (the thigh bone or the femur) is simply sitting on top of the other one (the shin bone or the tibia). The kneecap (patella) rests on the femur.

The knee joint happens to be the major weight-bearing joint of the human body. The knee joint primarily is a hinge joint, i.e., it moves in one plane. It is very similar to a door that opens and closes. The knee joint bends (flexes) or straightens (extends). The ligaments that stabilize the knee in these movements are called anterior cruciate ligaments and posterior cruciate ligaments that are attached to the femur and the tibia.

There is also a slight amount of rotation at the knee joint. This happens when you are getting on or off your bike, getting into or out of your car, etc. There are inner-side (medial) and outer-side (lateral) C-shaped discs called menisci that not only stabilize the knees during the rotational forces and reduce friction during movement, but also help in absorbing the pounding that the knee takes while walking and running.

Each of these bones have a protective coating (cartilage), allowing cushioning between the bones. The cartilage also allows for smooth gliding of the bones on top of each other when the knee moves, thus reducing friction. Also, from the inside, it is covered with synovium which secretes fluid to lubricate the joint and provide nourishment.

The 'Vastly' Ignored Muscle

As the name 'quadri' suggests, there are four components of the quadricep muscles. Two of them balance each other out, as one forms the outer portion (vastus lateralis) of quadriceps, whereas the other forms the inner portion (vastus medialis). Quadriceps are located in front of the thigh or the femur. All four components join together to form the common insertion tendon that attaches to the kneecap (patella). It further carries on as patellar tendon and finally attaches to the sharp bony prominence on the tibia, just below the knee joint.

If the inner portion of quadriceps (vastus medialis) is weaker than the outer portion, which almost always happens, courtesy long hours of sitting, it leads to muscle imbalances. Since quadriceps cross the hip and the knee joint, an imbalance of quadriceps causes a strain on both the knee and the hip joints; this can lead to an injury. Surprisingly, even in good athletes and sportspeople, this muscle is either weak as a whole or there is a major muscle imbalance.

The quadriceps straighten the knees, and also prevent them from buckling, hence they become very important in rehabilitation in case there is a ligament tear.

Hamstring Muscles Are at the Back of the Thigh

These back thigh muscles balance out the quadratus femoris. They begin at the sitting bones or the two prominent pointy bones that you sit on. You might feel them even if you have a well-cushioned bottom. They go and attach on both sides (inner and outer aspect) of the femur above and also below the knee joint.

Sitting for long hours, especially with a poor posture, shortens this muscle, effectively either putting it in a state of hyperactivity even at rest or making it go to sleep even when it should be working. Either way, they put too much pressure on the lower back, pulling it down, and not letting the knee straighten fully even while standing.

The Big Buttocks Muscle

Gluteus maximus is the big buttocks muscle, the one that we sit on. It is the one that gives shape to our bottom. Of course it has a far more important role than aesthetics alone. We don't realize that if we keep sitting on our two hemispheres, we'll soon become a sphere!

Gluteus maximus pulls the thigh back and rotates it out. It also stabilizes the hip joint. This muscle is very important for the lower back as well as for knee function. It is always taken for granted because many are not aware that it can also be used to correct the flat arches of your foot.

Self-assessment:

a. Stand up barefoot.
b. Don't bother about the correct posture.
c. Put your hands on your buttocks.
d. Now imagine there is a coin between your buttocks and you need to hold it tight so it doesn't fall off.
e. Tighten (contract) your bottom even more.
f. Now relax and do that again.
g. This time when you contract, notice what happens to the inside arches of your feet. You'll notice they begin to rise as you start to contract your buttocks muscles.

h. Hold that for 3 to 4 seconds.
i. Repeat twenty times. Do five sets throughout the day.

Psoas with a Silent P

The psoas is a very important core muscle that many are not aware of. It starts from deep inside the abdomen. To be precise, it starts from the front aspect of the lower spine, the area you would see if you were to remove your six packs, intestines and stomach. Effectively, it sits on either side of the centre of gravity of your body.

During walking or running, it is the psoas that raises your femur up. It gently rocks the centre of gravity of the body from one side to the other. When other muscles don't play their part properly, there would be too much swing with each step, leading to injuries in the ankles, knees, hips or the back.

The psoas muscle, therefore, is a very powerful flexor of the hip. It goes and attaches to the upper portion of the thigh bone (femur).

When you've been sitting for a long time, it becomes a habit for these muscles to acquire a shortened position and become very weak. This leads to back pain, knee pain and even foot pain because of excessive pressure with each step because the psoas isn't able to do its job properly.

As much as strengthening and stretching is important for psoas, it starts with you becoming more aware of it. Try to think of it while going about your daily work and notice the movements such as walking, jumping or getting up.

Classic Recipe for Disaster: Overpronating Charlie

Broadly speaking, your Charlie Chaplin stance, whether while sitting or standing, rotates your femur outwards at the hip joint. This leads to the hips going majorly out of alignment. Even though this would limit the hip's rotational movements, the hips will not start complaining till a lot later as it's a ball-and-socket joint. The outside of the quadratus femoris muscle (vastus lateralis), along with the ilio-tibial band, is overworked, whereas the inside of the quadratus (vastus medialis) is underworked and becomes very weak. This outside pull from muscles is initially an effect of poor posture while sitting, but soon contributes to the bad posture.

On the other hand, overpronation of the feet will make the shinbone (tibia) rotate inwards while walking and even more so while running. Again, the foot is designed in a way that it can handle inward and outward rolling, so it can take that for a while before complaining about it, unless, of course, there is a sharp twist, which can tear the ligament.

Both these conditions are common and very often coexist. This leads to excessive torsional force around the knee as the thigh muscle is being rolled out but shin bone is being rolled in. Soon, this ends up being a bit too much for the knee which primarily moves like a door, i.e., bending and straightening in one plane alone.

Diagnosis of Knee Pain

Very similar to back pain and contrary to popular belief, (osteo) arthritis isn't the commonest cause for knee pain. As a matter of fact, the cause for knee pain may or may not be primarily in the knee itself. Factors such as functionality of the legs, modern lifestyle leading to muscle imbalances and mal-alignments, along with sudden overuse and wearing mismatched shoes, whether running or formal footwear, all contribute to the underlying cause of most knee pains.

Let us look at knee pain based on the location of the pain, broadly dividing it into the front of the knee, the outer side of the knee, the inner side of the knee and the back of the knee.

Anterior or Front Knee Pain

Most knee pains are in the front and inner side of the knee. All this occurs because of overpronation at feet, muscle tightness, muscle weakness, problems in training, decreased hip mobility, inner thigh tightness, ilio-psoas tightness and restricting the movement in the hip and the knee.

A tight hamstring and gastrocnemius can cause the patella (kneecap) to be pulled outwards and hence change the biomechanics.

Patello-femoral Syndrome and Patello-femoral Tendinopathy

The above mentioned conditions are the most common causes for pain in front of the knee.

Their clinical features are similar, so differentiating between the two is difficult. Both conditions may occur simultaneously as a result of the same biomechanical abnormality or because of overuse or one may occur first and predispose the other. Repetitive activities such as basketball, long jumps, and high jumps may cause tendon irritation.

If front knee pain occurs at the beginning of an activity and settles down with warming up and returns after the activity, it could be patello-femoral pain syndrome.

Anterior Cruciate Ligament (ACL) Tear

Anterior cruciate ligament (ACL) tear is a common knee injury. Even though ACL injury is thought to be a sports-related (football, hockey, etc.) injury, it is also common among the non-sporting population. It can happen when one misses a step while running and suddenly trips. A classic complaint is having a sense of giving way or unstableness, whether it is a partial or full thickness tear.

Conservative treatment, involving a proper rehabilitation programme, is very important. In sports like football, hockey, etc., where there is a higher risk of an ACL injury, preventive programmes should be incorporated in training itself.

ACL reconstructive surgery is said to be the best treatment for an ACL tear. Orthopaedics the world over often assure their patients that 90–95 per cent of the time they would have a good to excellent result after the surgical intervention.[6] However, recent studies have shown that only 55–65 per cent of patients have been able to go back to their previous levels of activity or play after ACL reconstruction.[7]

These studies have highlighted that success of a surgery shouldn't only be limited to post-operative knee stability alone. It should be measured by return to the previous level of play or activity. Repeat injury of the recovered/operated knee and a risk of injury to the other knee should also be taken into account.

Patients need to be more aware of the latest scientific research in order to make informed decisions related to their treatment.

Each week, I see over half a dozen patients who have either had a second rupture of ACL after getting an ACL reconstruction by the top names in the game, or haven't been able to get back to playing at their previous levels of activities, whether it is sports or daily life. It bothers me immensely as something is definitely not right. Young active people, for whom their sport (football, Frisbee, cricket, basketball, etc.) is a big part of their lives, do everything right, from going to the doctors as soon as possible after the injury, getting all the possible investigations being asked for and then getting surgeries done by the top surgeons. They are great patients too when it comes to following advice on rest and rehabilitation. What is going on here? It would be too easy to put the blame on luck.

I am going to be unapologetic about my comments below because I am going to back up everything I state with facts. These are facts based on latest medical research published in top medical journals, especially the *British Journal of Sports Medicine (BJSM)*. They are not simply based on my opinions.

ACL rupture is not a simple injury. It has consequences that might mess up your future plans if not managed properly. ACL injuries lead to muscle weakness, functional deficits, lower sports participation, increased risk of repeat knee injury, and knee osteoarthritis. There is also a higher probability of getting meniscus injury, which further raises the chance of getting knee osteoarthritis in the future.

The point I am trying to make is that we need to recognize the importance of the correct management of an ACL injury. Something intense needs to be done. Does that mean you need to opt for surgery?

A Swedish study[8] published online first in the *BJSM* looked at a total of seventy-eight football clubs with 4,443 individual players from the highest national leagues in sixteen countries. They were followed over a varying number of seasons from January 2001 to May 2015 (365 club seasons and 10,157 player seasons were included for this analysis). I am using these numbers to make a point that what I am going to say next isn't coming from thin air, or based on a study conducted on a small sample of people.

This study, done over fifteen years, found that the return-to-play, at the same level three years later, as before the surgery, was only two-thirds after ACL reconstruction, i.e., 65 per cent. These were top players in the world, with access to the top surgeons. There was all the possible intention to get these players back on their feet because there was a lot of money riding on them. Yet, 4 per cent of them re-ruptured their ACLs even before the rehabilitation period was over.

So, what went wrong?

'Five to ten years ago, it was common for orthopaedic surgeons to assure their ACL injured patients that 90–95 per cent of the time they would have good to excellent results with surgical reconstruction. We suspect that such advice can still be heard in orthopaedic offices.'[9]

My patients tell me that this is true even today.

I believe that even with good intentions, if you are raising expectations of the patient, despite knowing otherwise, this qualifies as a lie. The dean of a renowned (liberal arts) university once told me that this is called marketing. I find that statement unbecoming of any human being; leave alone a professional of any kind.

A Norwegian study[10] published online first in the *BJSM* found that 30 per cent get injured again in the first two years of returning to previous level of activity/sports after ACL reconstruction. A study[11] published in January in the *American Journal of Sports Medicine* found a 7 per cent failure after the ACL reconstruction surgery. It also found that there was a 8 per cent risk of injury to the other uninjured knee as well. This total risk of 15 per cent (7 per cent plus 8 per cent) jumps to a 23 per cent failure rate for athletes under the age of twenty five.

Interestingly, players who returned to sports within nine months of surgery, and with more symmetrical quadriceps strength, markedly reduced their repeat injury rate.[12]

I am glad that I get mad at my ACL patients and therapists when I don't see their quadriceps to be up to the mark, even though their pain is better.

I also make a very simple point to my patients: 'Do they only want to play or run for a few more times and never again, or for life?' If the answer is for life, I tell them that they will have to stick to my timelines for rehabilitation to go back to their previous levels of activity. Surprisingly, most of them comply, even though they are most likely to be Type A personalities. It probably is because I am myself a Type A personality or because they know I run a 100-odd km at the drop of a hat even though I have a couple of disc bulges.

Time is a great healer but only if you do something appropriate with it. Appropriate rehabilitation becomes very crucial. Don't rush, because the injury might come rushing back.

To think a little beyond, ACL preventive programmes should be mandatory for athletes involved in sports where there is a higher risk of ACL injuries.

To sum it up, I will quote Don Shelbourne, father of accelerated rehabilitation, from a *BJSM* podcast.[13] He has performed more than 6,000 ACL reconstructions since 1982:

> Patients prefer a bit of instability with full range of motion than a stable knee. Stiff knee is a time bomb for osteoarthritis. Many surgeons overlook the loss of

motion as a risk factor. If you are wondering whether to have surgery or not after ACL injury—go for (appropriate) conservative management first.

Case (in her own words): Ira Leinonen, forty years old

I had an ACL injury twenty-two years ago while playing soccer. I was told I needed surgery. My teammate had gone through the same surgery and was not in a better position even after nine months. I was told that I was never going to play sports again; I was eighteen then. I didn't lose hope. After researching, I rehabilitated my knee by a series of stability and strength exercises. Twenty-two years on, during which I have regularly done kick-boxing, where jumping and landing on the knee is a common practice, my knee is holding on pretty well. I still follow my rehabilitation exercises on a regular basis. I plan to go on with the active lifestyle till the very end of my life.

Other Causes of Anterior Knee Pain

Stress fracture of the patella, quadriceps tendinopathy, patello-femoral instability, etc.

Pain in the Outer Aspect of the Knee

Ilio-tibial Band (ITB) Friction Syndrome

A very common reason for pain on the outside of the knee is ilio-tibial band friction or the ITB syndrome. Most of the times even good doctors and physiotherapists can get it wrong if they don't know enough about running. It is a common problem among long-distance runners.

This injury occurs with increased friction of ITB against the bony prominences at the outer lower end of the femur (thigh bone). The pain occurs while running when the knee passes through fifteen to thirty degrees of bending. It is usually around these angles that the foot strikes the ground while running and the person complains of outer knee pain. Downhill running worsens the situation as it reduces the knee flexion (bent) angle further. When more pressure is put on the knee, there is pain above the joint line on the outer aspect of the knee.

To start with, pain is felt on the outside of the knee after having run a certain distance and goes away with rest. However, at a later stage, pain can stay all the time and not improve with rest.

The usual reason for this to develop is inappropriate training involving sudden increase in mileage and speed running, overpronation, muscle imbalance, poor biomechanics and inappropriate shoes.

History and examination are usually ample and no investigation is needed.

To manage such cases, deep tissue release, stretching of tight structures like outer thigh muscles, hip rotators and calves, strengthening of weak muscles (vastus medialis oblique/inner portion of quads, inner thigh muscles and buttocks muscle) are very important. Wearing correct shoes at times can also solve the problem.

In extremely rare cases, use of corticosteroid injection or surgical release of ITB and excision of bursa may be required if conservative management has failed.

Lateral Meniscus Abnormality

The lateral (outer) meniscus injury is far less likely than the medial (inner) one. Sudden twist or trauma to the outside of the knee, e.g., while playing football, can lead to tear of lateral menisci. A worn-out lateral meniscus can present with a painful or non-painful bump at the above-mentioned site.

The onset of pain is gradual and localized to outer joint line—outer aspect of the knee where the thigh bone (femur) sits on the shin bone (tibia).

MRI can be done to confirm the diagnosis, if need be.

Osteoarthritis of the Outer Aspect of the Knee (Lateral Compartment Osteoarthritis)

Wear and tear of the outer aspect of the knee joint at the thigh (femur) and shin (tibia) bone occurs in conjunction with lateral meniscus injury.

Usually, there is increased pain after activities and stiffness after rest or sleep along with night pain with disturbed sleep. Morning stiffness is also a common complaint in this case.

Strengthening exercises play a major role in addressing muscle imbalances to rectify poor biomechanics. This should be combined with ice packs and NSAIDS for pain relief. Injections like corticosteroids and hyaluronic acid supplements (intra-articular) are useful. If appropriate conservative treatment fails, surgery such as TKR (total knee replacement), may be resorted to, but not rushed into.

Biceps Femoris Tendinopathy

Biceps femoris is the outer part of the hamstring muscle. Excessive acceleration or deceleration activities such as sprinting while playing football or hockey and excessive knee-bending exercises can cause the inflammation and degeneration of tendinous insertion of this muscle. Pain may also be felt due to the lengthening of hamstring muscle, e.g., when someone is trying to pull his shoe off the affected side using the other leg. The hamstring muscle is usually tight along with a stiff lumbar spine and deactivated gluteus maximus. It settles with rest and occurs again after activity.

Ultrasound is the investigation of choice for confirming the diagnosis.

Tendinopathies are usually treated by stretching and eccentric strengthening of the affected muscle. Rest and massage can be helpful initially.

Superior Tibial–Fibular Joint Injury

Besides the shin bone (tibia) there is another bone on the outside of the lower leg. It's called fibula. Tibia and fibula are joined just below the knee and then just above the ankle joint. The upper tibial–fibular joint can get injured as a result of direct trauma. It is also associated with rotational knee and ankle injuries.

Activities like pivoting and cutting demand tibial rotation and create pain. There is pain because of the direct pressure over the joint and altered joint movement, i.e., reduced or excessive movement on the joint.

Treatment mainly includes mobilization, strengthening and electrotherapy. Excessive mobility of the joint can be difficult to treat. Strengthening the surrounding structures is crucial. Local corticosteroid injections may help. Sometimes surgery has to be done in case of no symptomatic relief.

Referred Pain

Referred pain is a dull ache that is localized around the outer knee and can be referred from the lower back (lumbar spine) because of the irritation of the corresponding nerve.

Pain in the Inner Side of the Knee

Patello-femoral Syndrome

It is the most common cause for pain in the front and inner side of the knee as discussed earlier.

Medial Meniscus Abnormality

Tear or strain around the medial meniscus may also cause medial knee pain. The pain due to medial meniscus abnormalities is associated with certain twisting activities such as getting in or out of the car, getting on or off the bike, etc.

Case: Madhav Kumar, twenty-four years old

Madhav Kumar twisted his right knee a few weeks before he was supposed to join the Indian Army's Officers Training Academy in Chennai. For the twenty-four-year-old, this was a big blow—he had wanted to join the army for as long as he could remember. A scan revealed a tear in the medial meniscus. The knee was swollen, painful and stiff. A surgery was recommended, but that would prevent Kumar from joining the programme—in a month's time he was expected to run 2.5 km in 9 minutes, followed by a 25-km cross-country race that had to be completed in less than 3 hours.

Was there a way out for Kumar? Yes—three weeks of intense physical therapy not just to rehabilitate the knee, but also to correct other muscular imbalances in the body, and learning a running technique that would put less pressure on the knees. Kumar was sceptical at first, but gave in since this seemed like the only option. In two weeks, he was almost on his way to recovering full fitness. The last week was spent on running technique, on reducing his stride length without affecting the speed. At the end of the month, Kumar passed the physical examination and joined the academy.

Pes Anserine Tendonitis

The combined insertion of the three muscles (sartorius, gracillus and semitendinosus) on the inner side of the tibia, at the knee joint, is called pes anserinus. Inflammation of pes anserine tendon is under-diagnosed but common. It becomes inflamed as a result of overuse in swimmers, cyclists or runners. There is localized tenderness and swelling. Active contraction or stretching of the hamstring muscle causes pain.

Medial Collateral Ligament (MCL)

MCL (ligament at the inner aspect of the knee joint) sprain or bursitis does not occur as a result of any history of major trauma. Constant overpronation (rolling in of the foot) because of muscle imbalance and shoe–foot mismatch may cause an MCL strain.

Other causes of pain in the inner aspect of the knee are degenerative changes around the medial compartment of knee, referred pain from the lumbar spine or hip joint.

Pain in the Back of the Knee

Pain in the back of the knee can develop either gradually due to some underlying problem or due to some sudden injury. There can be a number of causes for pain in the back of the knee. The commonest ones are listed below.

Biceps Femoris Tendinopathy

Biceps femoris is a part of the hamstring muscle—a muscle located at the rear of your thigh. Its inflammation can lead to pain behind the knee, at the site of its attachment there.

This injury commonly happens with excessive acceleration and deceleration activities such as sprinting or in kicking sports like football, where a sudden, forcible contraction of the muscle happens.

Symptoms may include pain and tenderness around the attachment of the muscle behind the knee.

Immediate treatment can be ice compression, non-steroidal anti-inflammatory drugs (NSAIDs) and soft tissue release of the tight muscles.

Once the tendon starts to heal, strengthening the thigh and leg muscles is the mainstay of treatment.

Popliteus Tendinopathy

This is an injury to a small muscle located at the back of the knee. Its function is to provide stability and unlock the knee during initial bending.

Popliteus tendinopathy can be a result of overstretching or overuse of the popliteus, especially during downhill running.

The patient would feel pain while fully straightening the knee joint or during deep squats.

Treatment involves rest, icing with compression and the use of NSAIDs. Later, strengthening of the weak muscles surrounding the knee joint can be done.

Popliteus Bursitis or Bakers Cyst

Popliteus bursa is a fluid-filled pouch at the back of the knee. Its inflammation is known as popliteus bursitis, which can be caused either by a direct hit or because of overstrain to the knee.

Symptoms present themselves due to compression of adjacent structures. In this case, you will find a swollen, very tender mass that is size of a golf ball, palpable behind the knee joint.

Treatment involves icing, withdrawal from strenuous activities and NSAIDs. If symptoms persist for a few months, aspiration of fluid may be required.

Gastrocnemius Tendinopathy

The calf is made up of two muscles. The one that originates from above the knee joint is called gastrocnemius.

An inflammation or tear of this muscle can lead to posterior knee pain. The most common cause can be overuse, uphill running or if there is rapid increase in the mileage.

In this condition, jumping, hopping and calf raises would give immense pain behind the knee. Local tenderness will be present on pressing the injured area.

Initial treatment includes relief of pain and swelling by giving it rest and ice application. Depending on the extent of injury, a heel raise can be given if walking becomes too painful. Some soft tissue release and gentle stretching can be started soon after the injury.

If it's a minor injury, strengthening exercises like heel raises and heel drops can be started after 24 hours.

Radiating Pain from the Lower Back

Nerve root compression in the lumbar spine (lower back) can also cause pain behind the knee. Pain can also be felt due to the entrapment of nerves in the buttock region or behind the knee.

This results in pain radiating down the leg up to the knee or to the sole of the foot. Numbness and tingling sensation can also be associated with it which explains the neural disturbance.

Treatment of the back and relieving the compression of nerve with soft tissue releases, acupuncture, strengthening of core and back muscles and a few flexibility exercises can help in relieving knee pain.

Posterior Cruciate Ligament (PCL) Strain

PCL strain is not a common cause for pain in the back of the knee. It starts behind the knee and runs forward to attach to the front of the knee. Its function is to hold the thigh bone over the leg bone and prevent its displacement.

An injury to this ligament happens when there is direct blow to the leg leading to the overextension of the leg, like while playing football or if a person falls on the fully bent knee, common in downhill skiers.

The patient complains of poorly defined pain at the back of the knee with minimal swelling. Also there will be a feeling of instability in the knee joint.

Deep Vein Thrombosis (DVT)

Pain in the back of the knee because of deep vein thrombosis is not common but is very important to be aware of as it can be fatal if not managed properly and on time.

DVT is a clot of blood in the vein of the calf which can be the result of prolonged immobilization or post-surgery. It presents as calf pain or sometimes as pain behind the knee. It is important to diagnose it properly because if it is misdiagnosed, it can lead to serious injury or death. It can be confirmed by Doppler test or venography.

Osteoarthritis of the Knee

I have saved this one for the last for a specific reason. As mentioned earlier, there is a misconception that knee pain is because of knee arthritis (osteoarthritis). It is important to understand that basics need to be looked at before dealing with knee arthritis.

Osteoarthritis can cause pain medially, laterally and also in the front. There is wear and tear and changes in the knee joint. Initially, the pain is on activity, then at rest, and eventually increases at night too.

Knee replacements today are being done too often when not needed, and too soon, even if they are needed. Keep one very basic fact in mind: At the end of the day, it is your muscles that move you. Get them to start working. Your body will thank you for having taken this decision.

Case: Charles Mark[14] (name changed), fifty-three years old

A fifty-three-year-old, six-foot-tall man, weighing 146 kg, came to us with a left-knee pain; he had been experiencing this for over a year. His job involved very long hours of sitting. Of course weight had contributed to the problem by putting pressure on the knees, but we couldn't tell him to lose weight. That would have just added to his problems. Standing for as little as 5 minutes would increase his pain and stiffness. Upon examination, an orthopaedician told him that there was excessive soft tissue (menisci) injury, which was also confirmed on MRI. On having consulted me, he was told that he first needed to do strengthening exercises before deciding on surgery.

His treatment involved soft tissue release of tight and shortened muscles and strengthening and stretching exercises for various muscles. This was done to get grossly deactivated muscles to start moving again. This has made it easier for him to correct his posture as well. From the third week on, core muscle exercises were also incorporated. He did his exercises at home religiously. He was also advised 15–20-minute walks from the fourth week onwards, very unlike most treatment plans.

After six weeks of guided and supervised stretching, strengthening and conditioning, he reported a huge difference in the way he performed daily activities. He was much more confident and was able to go about his life without pain and stiffness. Small activities such as sitting, standing for long periods, walking and climbing stairs became easier. He now feels no morning stiffness. On the contrary, he feels very agile. Without getting any surgery, he has managed to reclaim his old life.

Patient's Testimonial: Himanshu Pattnaik, Badminton—Knee Injury

It was a fine Saturday morning of August 2010 and everything was going great till I lost consciousness and later found myself lying on the bench of the DDA sports complex indoor stadium in Dwarka. The last thing I remember was jumping for a smash and landing on an uneven floor, on the second court from the right, and twisting my knee. I cried in pain and felt like the lower portion of my leg had got separated from my left knee. I slowly opened my eyes to check if I still had my leg intact. Luckily it was, and I was convinced that I had messed it up big time.

Not knowing what to do, my well-meaning friends dropped me home. I was only able to stand with one leg, and the immediate thing that came to my mind was to see a doctor. I visited a nearby hospital and they said it was nothing alarming and could be a sprain and asked me to take a painkiller and wrapped a crepe bandage and let me go. I came home with the hope that everything was fine. However, I was not fully convinced because I was not able to walk without support and the pain was severe.

After struggling in pain for two days, I visited another orthopaedician (he had been great while treating my multiple wrist and fingers fracture two years ago) at one of the renowned hospitals in Gurgaon. He recognized me as we had built up a rapport during my earlier injury. The outcome of the interaction was shocking! He explained it had something to do with ACL (anterior cruciate ligament) and drew some picture to explain it to me in detail. Ten minutes later I was lying in a stretcher and he brought a syringe to take out some fluid from the knee joint for testing. When I demanded to know what was going on, he explained that he wanted to test (don't remember the test name) and suggested a knee surgery. He also explained that without the operation, I would never be able to play any kind of sport which involved movement in my life. I still remember that day vividly because I was scared to death. For a person like me, it was equivalent to pronouncing a death sentence. I almost ran out of the hospital fearing that he would operate if I stayed there any longer! I prepared myself to go through the knee operation, because sports is an integral part of my life.

I was depressed and afraid for my life. There were three things in particular which bothered me a lot: that I would not be able to participate in any sports activity, that I would not be able to ride my bike again and that I would not be able to play with my little angel (two-month-old daughter). In desperation, I reached out to friends I knew who had gone through similar experiences or those friends who were doctors, including in homeopathy, to see if there was any option other than surgery that would work out for me.

Finally, God heard my prayers. While interacting with a friend, he insisted I visit a particular doctor. I was not very keen to meet yet another doctor who would recommend surgery but I finally gave in to his insistent demands and decided to visit Dr Rajat Chauhan of Back 2 Fitness. I decided to try my luck. The clinic was far from Dwarka. However, by now I was eager to meet someone who could potentially help me. My friend got me an appointment and informed me that it was difficult to get an appointment with the busy doctor, so I had to be there on time.

My friend reached the clinic almost at the same time as I did. The plush ambience of the reception made me wonder if this was a moneymaking spa or a serious treatment facility. We were shown into the doctor's room.

Suddenly a man appeared and introduced himself as Dr Rajat with a smile, probably the only occasion when I have seen him in his formal attire (he is usually in his running gear). I narrated the whole story of my injury, shared the earlier prescription with all the ACL drawings, X-rays and MRI scan reports, etc. He quietly heard my story but his body language suggested it was a minor injury and he was ready with his suggestions before I had even completed my narration. He nodded quietly and asked me to lie down on the wooden bed that was stationed at the back. He hadn't said anything negative about the injury yet, so I was filled with hope. He tested my knee with movements up, down and sideways, and asked for a few sit-ups to be done with the support of the wall. By now I was used to wearing the brass knee brace while walking. We came back to our chairs to have a further discussion. He was cool and composed and ready to provide his inputs.

'Nothing to worry' was his first sentence and this lifted up my spirits! However, I decided to lower my expectations. He told me that I had two options, either I could undergo the various tests advised by the doctors so far or I could believe him when he said that it was a case of 20–30 per cent ligament tear. He suggested that the only way to tackle this was to build up the thigh, calf and buttock muscles, and that my injury was fully curable. He said that surgery was unnecessary. Without raising my hopes too much, I asked if I would be able to run again? Would I be able to ride a bike? He nodded his head in affirmation! I felt an immense sense of relief and felt all my tensions drain away at that instance. He further said that there was no need for any medicine or injections. He suggested I remove the brass knee brace and do the recommended exercises. I felt happy with the professional approach. The suggested exercises were emailed to me.

During my next visit, Kunal Vashist (senior sports and musculoskeletal physical therapist) taught me the exercises to be practised at home. I have never looked back since then! I followed all the advice and participated in all the activities organized by Dr Rajat, including on social media, just to say thanks. If I meet anyone suffering from ACL injuries, I do not hesitate to recommend Dr Rajat to them. It is hard to imagine what I would have done if I had not gone to see him.

Treatment of Knee Pain

- Hot/cold fomentation
- Taping to correct patellar mal-alignment

- Strengthening of the weak muscles
- Releasing of tight soft tissue structures
- Stretching for tight muscles

Strengthening is an important part of treatment and if the pain is the limiting factor, design the strengthening programme or modify it such that exercises happen pain-free. Progress on to the next level of exercises only if you feel the previous load was easier to manage and happened with the correct technique.

Hip Pain

Hip Osteoarthritis

Throughout our life we use joints like the hip, knee and ankle for activities like walking, squatting, jumping, running, etc. However, for unknown reasons we experience faster degeneration in either side of the hip leading to arthritis of the hip joint. Hip osteoarthritis is a single joint mechanical wear and tear of articular surfaces causing cartilage loss, osteophyte formation (bony spikes), synovial hypertrophy (capsular swelling) and restricted mobility of the affected hip joint. This can also be presented with a history of previous bone injuries on the same side. Severe arthritis has to be dealt with a hip replacement surgery. A person has to be more than sixty years of age, along with the pre-surgery hip strengthening protocol to gain maximum benefit from the surgery.

Early detection and prevention are the most important steps towards dealing with this disorder. Ice packs, NSAIDs along with rest provide relief from inflammation. Once out of acute pain, efforts should be made to recreate mobility around the lumbar spine, hip and ankle joints. Assessing the tight and weak muscles around the hip, knee and ankle is very important to design the rehabilitation programme. The muscle imbalance should be corrected along with core strengthening exercises. Balance becomes an important element in total rehabilitation since it develops proprioceptors for better joint stability. A combination of strength and mobility of affected hip and surrounding areas not only improve the stage of degeneration but can also delay the need for surgery.

Case: Bindu Badshah[15], fifty-nine years old

Bindu Badshah, a fifty-nine-year-old woman, visited us in November 2009 with osteoarthritis of the right hip and back pain, which she had been suffering from for many months. Her goal was to resume a normal life including walking, climbing, sitting for long periods in a pain-free situation.

Upon examination, her right hip was found to have very limited and painful active ranges. Muscular balances around her back, hip and knee were poor. Balance and stability issues had started to surface and there was poor strength around her hip and back muscles.

The treatment was structured in such a way that the painful symptoms were first catered to and, later, focus was placed on mobility and strength building.

Soft tissue manipulation and manual therapy sessions, along with the activation of core muscles, were the treatment given in the initial few months. Badshah showed confidence in the treatment and was willing to make it more intensive. One month later, a thirty-five-minute strength-training session was added for her back, knee and hip. This approach of combining manual therapy with strengthening and flexibility carried on for one year, with an attempt at making the session more productive each time. There were days when she was not in the best position to perform. We told her that the pain was like a stock market graph where upward and downward spikes should be appreciated as short-term changes. We need to simply stick to the plan.

She underwent bone mineral densitometry test after a year and a half. Her doctor was glad to find out that the bone density of her right femur and pelvis had improved markedly. She was going for long walks (on London roads), conducting exhibitions, climbing stairs to go to tube (metro) stations, sitting for long hours, writing . . . everything she had dreamt of doing one day, pain-free!

She still visits us, not mainly because of pain but to get even better. It is also for the maintenance of her pain-free situation, and for keeping her body happy and strong!

Testimonial: Bindu Badshah—A 'Core' Part of My Life

I walked into Dr Rajat Chauhan's clinic with little hope in November 2009. I was fifty-nine and had been diagnosed with arthritis in my right hip two months earlier. For several months I had been in constant pain, which only became worse when I got up or sat down in a chair, walked up the stairs, or squatted on the floor. My bone doctor had given his verdict: You will soon need a hip replacement, the sooner the better. It is advisable to get yourself a walking stick and don't load your hip . . . which meant don't sit, stand or walk!

I was completely devastated. The euphoria of my first exhibition of paintings had turned to dust. My dream of developing my art and holding a solo exhibition was fast dissolving while a feeble old age beckoned in the not-so-distant future. But in my mind, heart and spirit I was *not* old, not feeble, and refused to give in. It was at this very time that a friend recommended meeting Dr Rajat for a consultation.

Here I was sitting opposite this interesting man with sparkling eyes who heard my diagnosis and proceeded to examine me. 'Nonsense,' he said at the end of it! 'Tell me what you want your functional life to be and together we will make it happen.'

'I want to be pain-free, paint through the day, continue with t'ai chi (which had been giving me a lot of pain so I had stopped after four years), travel, walk and climb mountains and live a normal life.'

His answer was simply, 'Yes, all this will happen.' 'Do you promise?' I asked, and he answered, 'Yes.'

This is my sixth (2015) year with the clinic. I have continued with my painting, have had two mini exhibitions, restarted t'ai chi after a gap of two years, travelled abroad, taken tubes, climbed stairs, walked, visited Ladakh, been tossed in Goa's monsoon sea and I am mostly pain-free. When there is a return of pain because I've overdone something, my therapist uses his magical combination of soft tissue therapy and (acupuncture) needles to instantly sort it out. He knows every inch of my body and knows exactly what needs to be done and when. He increases weights when needed, adds floor exercises when necessary and monitors my day-to-day activities.

Trochanteric Bursitis of Hip

A typical complaint of pain on the outer side of the hip, which gets aggravated by standing, walking or sleeping on the same side, can raise the doubt about trochanteric bursitis. A bursa is a collection of tissues under bony prominences or between the muscles for better shock absorption and can act as a lubricant to reduce the friction required for smooth muscle movement. Due to repeated abnormal pressure around the gluteus muscle tendons or an uneven leg length creating extra pull around one hip can lead to inflammation and swelling of the outer hip bursa (greater trochanteric bursa).

Even in the case of internal transport barriers syndrome, the involvement of the same musculature (gluteus maximus and tensor fasciae latae) can create a lot of friction to produce bursa inflammation. A poor biomechanics of the foot can increase lateral excursion on the pelvis leading to increased pressure on the greater trochanter resulting in a gradual inflammation. Lastly, a direct blow or injury around the greater trochanter can also be the cause. Understanding the root cause through proper history and assessment can help create a successful treatment plan.

In mild to moderate pain, controlling the inflammation through icing/NSAIDs along with activity modification is generally required. Tight muscles such as gluteus medius, quadratus lumborum, tensor fasciae latae, vastus lateralis and lattisimus dorsii should be released along with the stretching programme to regain flexibility. The exercise plan should include hip abductor/adductor strengthening, core strengthening, pelvic stability and correction of overpronation with shoe modification, if necessary. In severe pain, corticosteroid injection or removal of the inflamed section of the bursa is advisable.

FAI (Femoral Acetabular Impingement)

The hip joint is a ball-and-socket joint where the socket is made by one side of pelvic bone that sits over the ball of the thigh bone. An impingement of the hip joint occurs when the ball of thigh bone abnormally collides with the socket of the pelvis. This can occur either by excessive bone growth on the head of the femur/ball (cam deformity) or excess bone growth on acetabulum/socket (pincer deformity) or even both. This abnormal collision occurs in certain angles, leading to pain and limitation of mobility in the hip joint, majorly aggravated by standing and walking. At times, it is only a muscular imbalance caused by tightness around Ilio-psoas and adductor muscles ; this abnormally limit the hip mobility and pain. Finding the right cause can help in alleviating the symptoms. If not managed properly, this can lead to premature hip arthritis.

In all the possible causes, it is important to control pain through cold compression and anti-inflammatories and correct muscular imbalances to regain normal joint motion. Strengthening of core, hip and surrounding joints is very important to increase the success rate. Failed cases can be further referred for surgical correction of the femoral angle to minimize or solve the possible impingement with the aim of preventing premature arthritis.

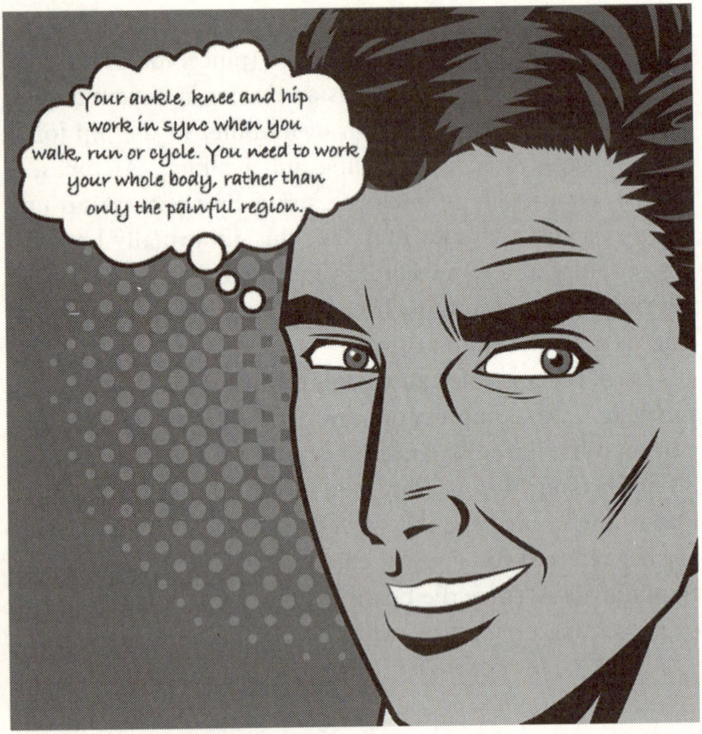
Your ankle, knee and hip work in sync when you walk, run or cycle. You need to work your whole body, rather than only the painful region.

8

OTHER COMMON ACHES AND PAINS[1]

Though I have focused on back pain throughout the book, it is important to also look at some common musculoskeletal conditions.

Fibromyalgia[2]

The diagnosis of fibromyalgia has evolved over the century—going through the labels of muscular rheumatism,[3] fibrositis, fibromyositis, myo-fibrositis and myo-fascial pain syndrome. Going by the various names, one can easily guess that the disorder has to do with inflammation of the soft tissues, i.e., muscles, ligaments, tendons and connective tissue. It is, in fact, the most common cause of widespread musculoskeletal pain in women (about 3 per cent) than in men (about 1 per cent). It is a disorder that often occurs first in people of working age and has a variable course after that; remitting completely in some and carrying on for decades in others.

There are several hypotheses about the causes of fibromyalgia ranging from genetic, neuro-endocrine (dopamine, serotonin), neuro-endocrine, neuro-inflammatory, lifestyle and psychological. It is a fact that fibromyalgia is more common in those with chronic fatigue syndrome, depression and anxiety disorders, whether they are causative or not.

It is important to distinguish fibromyalgia from other similar disorders and also to rule out the underlying medical conditions like hypothyroidism and other rheumatic diseases.

According to the criteria laid out by the American College of Rheumatology (ACR), a person is tested for fibromyalgia when he/she has widespread pain at predefined 'trigger points' for at least three months along with sleep disturbance, tiredness and weakness. The diagnosis is often made after ruling out other similar conditions and may require laboratory tests and consultation with mental health professional.

To treat fibromyalgia is to attack it from multiple sides all at once. Treatment may involve anti-depressants, anti-anxiety and anti-seizure medications along with psychotherapy, exercise, neuro-feedback and physical therapies like 'trigger point release' massage.

It needs a team of doctors and therapists to beat this 'gang' of symptoms. When looking for a specialist to treat fibromyalgia, pay attention to whether your specialist is a part of, or can work together with, a team of other physicians and therapists.

Neck Pain

Upper Cross Syndrome

The commonest cause for pain in the neck, upper back, shoulder and arms is actually not what most people are labelled by. It is the upper cross syndrome which is secondary to a sedentary sloppy lifestyle that we all lead, where we sit in a poor posture for very long hours. No matter what our occupations, all of us use smartphones, tablets, laptops and desktops for very long hours. Muscles initially respond to it as a protective mechanism, but over time it becomes second nature.

Upper trapezius, levator scapulae, sternocleidomastoid and pectoral muscles become tight whereas the deep neck flexors and lower stabilizers of the shoulder blade (serratus anterior, rhomboids, middle and lower trapezius) become deactivated (weak).

This leads to a typical forward-positioned head along with elevated and forward-positioned shoulders. This position stresses the top of the neck, the junction where the neck (cervical vertebra) joins the upper back (thoracic vertebrae) spine, and the area in between the shoulder blades (fourth thoracic vertebra). It also stresses the shoulder joint and reduces the joint's stability. This alters the movement in the neck, the shoulders and the upper back.

This posture also limits chest expansion during deep breathing. Eventually, it alters the whole body's movements, including the gait. This ends up being a predisposing factor for pains in the upper body that then go misdiagnosed for a very long time.

Investigations aren't very useful in upper cross syndrome. A skilled therapist or doctor will be easily able to pick up on it. The ones not experienced in it might order for a battery of tests and could be misled by any findings that the sensitive investigations pick up.

Usually manual therapy by osteopaths, chiropractors or physiotherapists is useful, but not for the long term. Sometimes, the benefits might only last a few hours. Similarly, posture correction sounds great in theory, but on its own it doesn't last for very long unless the muscle imbalance is taken care of. Appropriate exercises on a regular basis are very important to address the muscle dysfunctions and movement patterns for long-term results. This involves strength training, stretching and functional movements. If the daily triggers, like excessive usage of smartphones and computers, are not limited, it's only a matter of time before the symptoms come back. There needs to be a major lifestyle change.

Cervical Lock Syndrome

Patients often come with a very stiff neck, almost locked. Most of the time, nothing in particular has triggered it. They could have simply woken up with a very stiff neck which is very painful to move. At times, sudden but simple movements like turning your neck cause it.

The pain is way out of proportion to how bad the condition actually is. Mostly, the bones go out of alignment, just slightly, leading to muscle spasms. It is important to not fight the pain.

Ice compression and anti-inflammatories, along with rest, tend to do the trick. It might last a couple of days. It's important to not push pain or go back to excessive intense physical activity right away. Support your neck at night by placing a rolled up towel under your neck.

Cervical Spondylosis (CS)

This is an overused term like slipped disc for back and arthritis for knee pain. Most cases of neck pain have nothing to do with spondylosis.

Cervical spondylosis refers to degenerative changes of the cervical spine (neck). Terms like cervical osteoarthritis or neck arthritis are interchangeably used. Even when it does happen, poor lifestyle, poor posture while sitting, prolonged sitting and sleeping in a poor posture make matters worse.

Cervical spine (neck) is mobile but it is stacked upon the thoracic spine (upper back), which has limited mobility. Excessive movement restriction in the upper thoracic puts more pressure on the neck area.

It is important to gradually increase the strength around the upper back, stretch the pectoralis major muscles and keep moving the neck. The posture you keep throughout the day plays a very important role.

Follow these points to deal with cervical spondylosis:

- Don't sit for more than 30–45 minutes at a stretch.
- Limit the use of smartphones, tablets, laptops and computers. Even while using these gadgets maintain a good posture.
- Improve your posture throughout the day and night.
- Stretching, strengthening and maintaining a range of motions should become a part of your daily routine for the whole body.

Note: Some advices for sleeping and sitting postures have been discussed in earlier chapters, including spine mobility and strength exercises.

Cervical Disc Prolapse

Like spondylosis, cervical disc bulge and prolapse are over-diagnosed. Cervical (neck) disc bulge is very similar to the lumbar (lower back) bulge. When the bulging disc irritates the spinal cord, it could cause pain in the neck and pain, numbness and tingling sensation down the arm. The distribution of symptoms can suggest where the problem is.

The majority of the suffering population gets better through conservative management like through ice compression, anti-inflammatories, strengthening and mobility exercises along with following postural advice. Some people may need anti-inflammatory or corticosteroid injections at the affected cervical level along with conservative treatment.

Very similar to a lumbar disc bulge, injections or surgical procedures are rarely needed. Surgical procedures could range from partial discectomy to complete disc removal with fusion or artificial disc replacement.

Shoulder Pain

Rotator Cuff Tendinopathy

The rotator cuff is a group of four muscles (supraspinatus, infraspinatus, teres minor and subscapularis) which, as the name suggests, cuff around the ball (head of humerus) of the shoulder joint. These muscles stabilize and control the shoulder and help in rotational movements.

The inflammation of these muscles is called rotator cuff tendinitis. It's a common cause of shoulder pain and impingement in athletes. In this, patient complains of pain with overhead activities like throwing a ball, swimming or any racquet sport like tennis, badminton, squash, etc.

The initial treatment includes rest, ice compression or, if pain still persists, maybe a corticosteroid injection. Rotator cuff and scapular strengthening exercises can help in relieving pain.

Shoulder Impingement

The rotator cuff tendons in the shoulders are protected by bones (mainly the acromion) and ligaments that form an arch over the top of the shoulder.

With age-related degeneration of these bones or the muscular imbalance around the shoulder joint, these rotator cuff tendons get intermittently trapped and compressed during shoulder movements. Hence, it leads to the impingement of the shoulder joint.

In this case, patients complain of swelling, pain and a restricted range of motion of shoulder joint.

Initial treatment of shoulder impingement is rest and NSAIDs. Once the pain settles down, rotator cuff and scapular strengthening exercises are the solution.

Anterior Dislocation

Dislocation of shoulder joint is one of the most common traumatic injuries. It is associated with acute trauma leading to sudden onset of severe pain and inability to move the arm. Pain is generally described as a feeling of the shoulder 'popping out'. There can be bruising with this injury. A compression fracture of the arm (humerus) bone may be present.

If you suspect a dislocated shoulder, don't try to move the joint and seek prompt medical attention. X-Ray is the investigation of choice.

Most people regain full shoulder function within a few weeks. However, once you've had a dislocated shoulder, your joint may become unstable and get prone to dislocations.

Frozen Shoulder/Adhesive Capsulitis

The common age during which adhesive capsulitis occurs is between forty and sixty years. It is not uncommon after some trauma, a fracture or a surgery of shoulder, arm or forearm. It affects the left shoulder more than the right and is more prevalent in women than in men. People with diabetes are prone to a frozen shoulder.

The history of stiffness in the shoulder makes it easy to diagnose this condition. The patient complains of difficulty in wearing clothes, combing hair and other overhead activities. Frozen shoulder is a self-limiting condition which resolves in two-and-a-half years. So, one option of treating it is to wait for it to resolve on its own.

Evidence suggests that physiotherapy, exercises, drugs and injections hasten the healing process and reduce recovery time.

Referred Pain

The joints of neck and upper back often refer pain to the shoulder and arm. In the younger population, referred pain can be a result of a disc herniation or an acute injury causing impingement of an existing nerve.

Disc herniation accounts for 20–25 per cent of the cases of cervical radiculopathy. In older patients, cervical radiculopathy is often a result of narrowing of the cervical joint space from bony degenerative changes and decreased disc height.

It is important to have the history to see if the patient experienced neck pain or stiffness, though, spine may refer pain to the shoulder and arm even when there is no local neck pain present.

Factors associated with increased risk include heavy manual labour, smoking and driving or operating vibrating equipment. Other, less frequent, causes include tumours of the spine.

Neural stretching might help in restoring the normal function of the neural structure.

An active trigger point in the shoulder and neck muscles can also refer pain to the shoulder.

Soft tissue release and trigger point therapy can help in reducing pain.

Biceps Tendinopathy

The head of the biceps, which is attached to the shoulder, is susceptible to shoulder injury. This commonly happens in athletes who do weight training regularly or do exercises such as bench presses and dips.

Symptoms include local tenderness and pain. Pain may increase because of stretching the biceps or by contracting the muscle against resistance.

Local application of NSAIDs and soft tissue release helps in relieving pain.

Fracture of Clavicle

It is the most common fracture seen in sporting activities. It is usually caused from a fall on the shoulder, for example, in horse riding, or cycling, or direct contact with opponent in sports such as football. It causes localized tenderness and swelling. An X-ray reveals the site of fracture.

Acromioclavicular Joint Injuries

This also happens with the fall on the point of shoulder. In this case, there is either injury to the capsule of the shoulder or maybe a partial or complete tear of the ligament of the shoulder attached to the same joint.

It is managed with immobilizing the injured part in a sling for several weeks depending on the extent of injury.

Elbow Pain

Tennis Elbow

Tennis elbow, also called lateral elbow pain, is a common injury found in racquet sport players such as badminton or tennis and in manual labourers like carpenters and plumbers. The most common cause is excessive wrist movement.

In this, pain is generally localized on the bony prominence of the outer aspect of the elbow joint, rarely spreading down to the forearm and wrist.

In sportspersons, it can be caused due to recent changes in training or technique or equipment used in sports. In the non-sporting population, it can happen due to repetitive wrist movement at work like in typing or writing. The pain is bad enough to stop you from playing or doing your work as sometimes it may aggravate with simple everyday activities like picking up a glass of water or shaking hands.

Rest, cold compression and over-the-counter painkillers often help relieve tennis elbow.

If pain persists, use of a brace or elbow strap gives good support to alleviate pain.

If your symptoms haven't improved after six to twelve months of extensive conservative therapy, you might have to get surgery to remove damaged tissue. These types of procedures can be performed through a large incision or through several small incisions. Rehabilitation exercises are crucial for recovery.

Golfer's Elbow

People with golfer's elbow or medial elbow pain, have pain on the inner aspect of the elbow joint.

Like a tennis elbow, it is not limited to golfers only. In this case, pain is related to excessive throwing activities. Repetitive throwing, especially when the throwing technique is poor, leads to the stretching of ligament and muscular tissues around the inner and front side of elbow joint, creating instability.

Patients complain of pain and tenderness around the inner aspect of the elbow joint. At times, the pain spreads to the forearm and wrist.

There can be stiffness around the elbow, weakness around the wrist and hand.

It usually responds to rest and ice compression for 5 minutes, three to four times a day.

Wrap your elbow with an elastic bandage or use a splint. You can take oral NSAIDs, like ibuprofen, naproxen, or aspirin to reduce the pain and swelling. You may also get an injection of a corticosteroid or painkiller (like lidocaine) in the elbow.

If this fails, surgery may be an option. The procedure involves minimally invasive, ultrasound-guided removal of scar tissue in the region of the tendon pain.

Wrist Pain

De Quervain's Tenosynovitis

It's an inflammation of the muscular attachments of the thumb, common in athletes like rowers, canoeists and golfers because of the way they hold their sport equipment.

In this condition, the thumb becomes tender and this worsens when a person makes a fist with his/her thumb inside. It can be so painful that the patient may not even be able to hold a pen.

Treatment includes splinting the thumb, resting, cold compression and avoiding activities that aggravates pain. Stretches and strengthening exercises are recommended.

Increasing the diameter of the pen by adding an extra rubber grip might help.

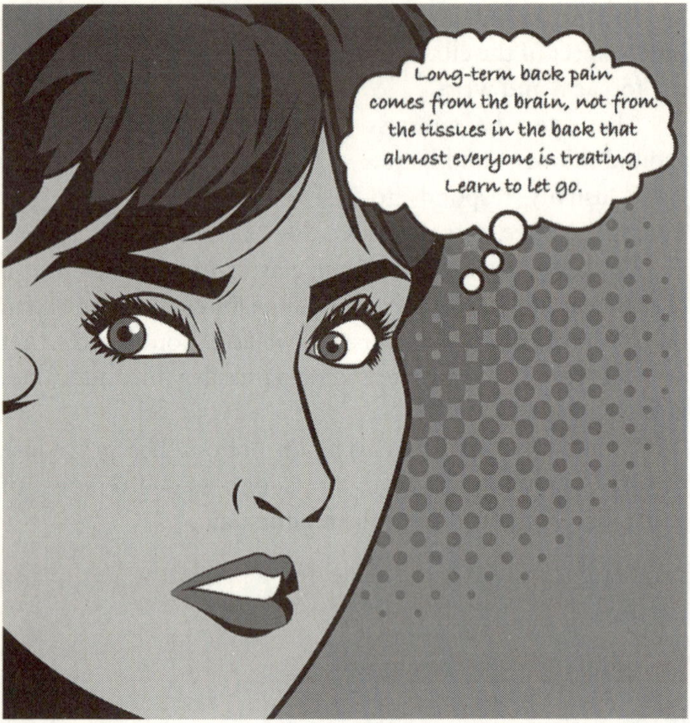
Long-term back pain
comes from the brain, not from
the tissues in the back that
almost everyone is treating.
Learn to let go.

9

PAIN IS INEVITABLE, SUFFERING IS OPTIONAL

'It is not what happens to us that determines our character, our experience, our karma, and our destiny—but how we relate to what happens.'[1]

Even though back pain seems to be the biggest bane of modern society, you have the power to change your condition. You might not be able to change your genes, but you can change how those genes are expressed with some effort. Along with regular physical activity and exercise, you need to alter eating habits and other lifestyle-related habits. Even before you were born, the conditions that would eventually lead to back pain were already being created in terms of your mother's calcium intake and exposure to sunlight. So, a passive approach won't work. You will have to make it happen.

'Regular (endurance) exercise decreases exercise-induced inflammation in humans while occasional exercise increases inflammation even more than not doing any exercise.'[2]

Modern society is one of the main reasons why back pain is such a big problem today.

The modern sloppy lifestyle offers a fertile ground for back pain to blossom. Super experts out there try to address the last straw on the camel's back, or in this case yours, without looking at the bigger picture. Somehow, instant relief is the order of the day—both for the sufferer and the healer. For a long-term solution, we need to understand the *why* rather than the *what*. For long-term management, lifestyles need to be understood and addressed.

> Back pain and its consequences are not isolated physical problems but are associated with other conditions such as social, psychological, and workplace-related factors. These factors—stress, worry and anxiety, along with the patient's own perceptions of and ability to manage the problem—can make the short duration back pain into a chronic one. The obvious role of both the society and psychology in this respect suggests that such factors should be considered an integral part of back pain in relation to preventive efforts, in the initial and later phases of treatment.[3]

Since there is no single reason for the ongoing long-term back pain, we need to look at the smaller things that add up. These need to be addressed. There is no formula, and there is no one-solution-cures-all either for back pain. Multiple small triggers need to be identified and addressed. Not one magical solution which is suggested by almost all.

Modern Lifestyles

It almost appears that technology advancement and physical fitness are inversely correlated. In a beautiful piece, Jared Diamond[4] made a convincing case for the discovery of agriculture being 'the biggest mistake in the history of the human race'. Why? Didn't everyone say that was the best thing that possibly happened to mankind? It's because it made you move as little as possible. Even though farming involves sowing seeds and maintaining the fields till the crops are ready for harvesting, the physical activity was a lot lesser than while being a hunter-gatherer. You had to hunt and gather the kill every few days if not every day. Compared to today, farming seems physically exhausting , but compared to the hunter-gatherer era, it seems sloppy. That was the beginning of us humans becoming lazy.

There are two sayings about this, one is popular but rarely practised, the other is not so popular but widely practised:

> Why lie down, if you can sit
> Why sit, if you can stand
> Why stand, if you can walk
> Why walk, if you can run.

The other one is:

> Never run when you can walk.
> Never walk when you can stand.
> Never stand when you can sit.
> Never sit when you can lay down.
> Never lay down when you can sleep.[5]

Which one do you think you practise more? Now don't feel embarrassed, you are not alone. Almost the entire world practises the latter. But don't think that if the majority practises something, it is right. You know better.

So, why did the shift from hunter-gatherer to agriculture happen? It was because of the good old ROI (return on investment) philosophy that Homo sapiens mastered.

We weren't made to be stationary and sitting on chairs in front of computer screens or televisions. In too short a span, less than a hundred years, there has been a massive technological leap which has led to drastic changes in our lifestyles. It has confused this amazing piece of machinery called the human body, which struggles to adapt to these rapid changes. This jet-set modern lifestyle is the primary cause for the back pain epidemic we see around us. No one owes us anything. It is not just about coming to terms with this reality but tackling it and being better prepared for dealing with it.

We were made to move, but today's lifestyle stops us from moving. A couple of decades ago, back pain was an issue for the elderly but today even children complain of chronic back pain. We need to make some major changes in our outlook and lifestyle to prevent this.

Who Is Responsible for Your Condition?

Back pain starts gradually and factors from the beginning of your life play a role in it. Only in very rare cases does it come on suddenly, out of the blue.

There are two sets of people responsible for back pain being such a big nuisance in all our lives.

The first person is you.

Second is anyone who has directly or indirectly contributed to the environment that you live in. This includes your parents, teachers, partners, employers and your children. The cycle of life goes on. These roles are important because you could also be in one of these positions, affecting someone else's life.

You, the Sufferer

In India, people rush to specialists with the minutest of problems. Back pain is a great example of this. In a majority of cases, simple back pain is easy to manage. Orthopaedicians or neurosurgeons are considered the final authorities on back pain in the traditional healthcare set-up. However, surgery is needed only in less than 2–5 per cent of all lower back pain cases. If surgery is not required, then surgeons are not equipped to address the situation. Since early on in their medical education and career, they focus on getting good at surgical procedures. Their forte isn't conservative management (non-invasive) of back pain. We all assume that they are authorities on the subject; from physiotherapy modalities like ultrasound, interferential and laser, to alternative treatments like acupuncture and massage, to lifestyle changes. Of course, this is not meant to be a negative criticism. There is only so much you can focus on. I focus on conservative management of back pain, for instance. I am not an expert at all the details of surgeries offered for back pain.

Does this confuse you as to what to do and whom to go to? Good. Confusion eventually leads to clarity, but for that you need to make the effort of knowing more. It's your body. It's your job to be better informed.

All of us, who are busy blaming everything and everyone else for our current status, need to accept our physical (un)fitness levels and change our mindsets. We need to take the onus and do something to change it. No amount of passive treatment in isolation, including surgery, will permanently fix the problem. It's important to realize that you aren't simply a piece of furniture that needs a nail or a screw in the right place. There is a lot more to it. Respect yourself.

Make yourself a priority. You need to get started, rather than waiting for someone else to solve your problem. After all, it *is* your problem.

Preschool (0–3)

Human babies begin to move from the time they are born. It is our basic instinct to move. We want to run even before we can stand unassisted. Babies can learn how to swim before they learn to walk. We simply love moving from one point to another. Sitting quietly in any one place for any length of time is counter-intuitive for us.

Nowadays, smartphones and tablet computers are handed to babies, even before they turn one, by parents who want to keep them quiet and not run around. Soon enough, they are put in crèches where they are made to sit and keep still; when they are supposed to be running about and exploring the world around them. To be fair, some crèches understand that, but most don't. When at home with parents, they are expected to sit quietly in a corner.

Unfortunately, it suits well-intended busy parents as their children sit in one place and don't need assistance. They don't realize they are changing them for life. It goes against nature. We were made to move. That was the norm a couple of decades ago but technology has played a major role in changing that aspect of society.

Seats in strollers and car seats for infants are actually poorly designed. They force young children to sit still in a poor posture. Poor posture is thus being imposed on children. What parents don't realize is that this will take a long time to correct in their adulthood.

Soon enough there is pressure to get children admitted to good schools, and 'discipline' and 'robotic' behaviour is encouraged. Moving, which comes naturally to us, is discouraged. In this way, without realizing, people who care for us the most lay the foundation for a lifetime of back pain.

Solution

As I reiterate throughout the book, it is important to realize that we are made to move. The first three years are the foundation years of our lives. Children should be allowed to play to make their physical foundation sturdy. This will enable them to take on problems like back pain and other chronic diseases that are lifestyle-related.

Outdoor activities, picnics with parents every weekend and annual vacations that involve physical activities should be encouraged.

In school too physical activity can't simply be confined to a senseless sports class and health can't be taught just to pass an exam. It's recommended to start from as early as three years of age, because that's when the education system starts dictating the lives of children. These days children as young as one-year-olds are sent to pre-nursery schools. It simply isn't natural to force a child that young to sit down, that too quietly, for long periods of time.

Pre-teen (4–12)

In my practice, I often see young kids suffering from posture and lifestyle-related backaches. Today children and youth have reflexes on computer games that can match that of fighter pilots, but these children are physically very unfit. They are worse than even adults three to four times their age.

By the age of three or four, when you have just about started school, you are forced to sit for a minimum of 4 to 6 hours, which is one-sixth to one-fourth of your day. Soon enough, it becomes 6 to 8 hours, i.e., a quarter to a third of your day. As much as the agriculture revolution made us sedentary, in today's modern world we are getting to a very different level of sloppiness. A quarter to a third of your life is spent sitting on poorly designed chairs and in poor postures.

To make matters worse, students are expected to wear shoes in schools and also at home. For almost half a day, their feet are encased in poorly designed and uncomfortable shoes. No shoe company seems to be interested in improving the design of these shoes because they are sold without making any effort. No one seems to be asking for better quality or comfort. It probably happens because neither are school-going children bothered about their school shoes, nor are their well-intentioned but ever-busy parents.

Even if the shoes were decently designed, you might consider that human feet have a high density of nerve endings, and wearing socks and shoes for half our lives ends up numbing them.

The spine is fragile at this age, but most schools make students carry heavy bags every day. Carrying the heavy weight of poorly designed school bags and the resultant poor posture leads to long-term damage to spines. It might not hurt right away, but it is irreversible.

The combination of all these factors—sitting for long periods of time, wearing uncomfortable school shoes, and carrying heavy school bags—ensures the weakening of those fragile backs of our next generation. Lifelong back pain just happens to be one of the by-products of modern schooling. Somehow, this doesn't bother too many decision makers who are busy creating educational institutions. However, it is a basic fact that the brain resides in a body. If the bodies are not able to live a long and healthy life, the minds too will not be able to work at their optimal levels.

If posture isn't addressed at this age, it becomes a lot more difficult to correct it later in life because brain patterns have been formed. This is true for movement as well.

Solution

Pre-teen years are the most neglected by parents when they actually are a child's foundation years. They play a vital role in the kind of individuals children grow up to be. During these years, children are neither babies nor are they adults. Probably because of that, they are almost taken for granted. Once in their teens, the mould has already set, both mentally and physically. They aren't ready to absorb and adapt as easily. Pre-teen age group is extremely impressionable. They soak a lot of what they see, hear and learn. A simple example is skiing. It comes naturally when learnt at a younger age but as one gets older, it keeps getting tougher to pick up skiing from the scratch.

Parents need to set an example, not just by preaching but also by practising. Children emulate what they see and pick up good habits without you making too much of an effort if they see you doing it. Parents need to regularly play sports and exercise. Also, parents have to make better food choices rather than giving them sweets and fast food as rewards. Your annual vacations need to be planned around physical activities rather than going to concrete jungles. The same applies to teachers as well.

Parents first need to stop spending time on gadgets such as smartphones, tablet computers, laptops, desktops and in front of the idiot box (television). That gives parents far more credibility to tell their children to do the same. In my own friend circle and patients I see, a growing number of them now don't have television sets in their homes. This creates a good environment which is just not about spending leisure time in front of the idiot box but being more physically active. Children should be encouraged to play outdoors rather than board games or computer games. Technology is today's reality, so it's fair to ration time spent on it rather than completely ban it, because that's not going to really work.

Sitting is a big nuisance too. Children need to study but that doesn't have to go hand-in-hand with sitting. There should be standing desks at home and even at school. I would suggest that students should be made to stand for at least two classes a day, or at least one class should be held outdoors.

I am not a big fan of standard school shoes, especially those black leather ones. Parents can probably request schools to either stop requiring children to wear these shoes or to allow children to take them off during classes. For schools and schoolteachers, the latter is a practical tip. When we come home, the first thing we all tend to do is kick off our shoes. It instantly relaxes us. Children should be made to do the same during back-to-back classes. They'll feel a lot more relaxed and will have a better posture too. This will help markedly reduce the pressure and stress on lower backs.

Another major factor that needs to be addressed to nip chronic back pain in the bud is the use of heavy, poorly designed school bags. This is one area where technology can definitely help in reducing the weight of school bags or getting rid of them completely. The government should invest in making tablet computers mandatory in schools and make the whole syllabus available online. Imagine having no books at all! That's where the world is headed. This will improve posture and put a lot less stress on young backs.

Physical education classes are a standard in all schools. Mostly they end up being senseless play sessions or no session at all, because the school focuses way too much on academics and considers physical education a waste of time, effort and resources. Rarely, courtesy passionate sports teachers or administration, do they offer sport-specific sessions. In all cases, fitness is almost always neglected.

Different aspects of health and fitness need to be integrated into all subjects being taught to this age group. Children are inquisitive by nature. They are keen to know the 'why' of everything. Once we can answer that, it becomes easier to make them do any activity for life. So physical education should be well-integrated with academics, and not just restricted to one class a week. In academics, the plan shouldn't simply be to teach so that students can pass an examination. Engage the students. Engage them with their parents and teachers. Only then will we make a bigger impact on society.

Getting children physically active and helping them make right food choices will make them a lot less prone to lower back pain and other chronic diseases. Schools should not use physical exercises and activities as punishments, as this leads to children attaching a negative connotation to them.

Case: Taruna Rai (name changed), twenty-three years old

A twenty-three-year-old came to me with lower back pain. She admitted that she wanted to pick up a sport but suffered from a weird fear—ballophobia, a term coined by her, which meant she was scared of anything that was thrown towards her, especially a ball or a Frisbee. This started from her early school days. The principal in her school was so particular about cleanliness that he had forbidden students from playing on the school campus. Can you even imagine that! Sadly, he affected a lot of lives being the principal of a popular school. This was when Taruna's ballophobia began.

This was a case that didn't need much technical know-how, but simply listening to her story led me to the solution. What was needed was some motivation to get her moving, rather than making a detailed exercise programme along with medication. She showed remarkable improvement. Today, she is a mentor to others like her who are reluctant to pick up a sport.

Even for the biggest problems, we just need to apply common sense but we are too busy complicating matters.

Teenage Years (13–20)

This age group is a rebel almost without a cause, or at least that's what we 'adults' think. To be fair, they are simply unsure and confused about their identity. They need our help but not our pity. The only way to help them understand is to empower them with knowledge and then let them decide, rather than force anything down their throats. It'll surprise us all but they are far more mature than the generations before them.

By the time children reach this age, they are already moulded both physically and mentally; so contrary to popular belief that a lot more effort has to be put in to enable them to make changes, whether to their bodies or their mindsets, we only need to nudge them in the right direction. The moment we force them, we lose the plot. We also need to appreciate that they have different priorities in life. At this age, the 'we-are-immortal' syndrome is at its peak. They don't appreciate investing in the future. It doesn't make sense to them to talk about leading a healthy lifestyle so that they can lead better lives later. This is the generation of instant gratification. Adults, who look for instant results, make the situation even worse.

Peer pressure plays havoc with their minds too. If their foundation in the early years wasn't solid, they'll have poor posture; will not be able to address the issue at this age because it is simply not a priority for them. To look cool is a lot more important than a good posture. As they grow taller and there are other physiological and anatomical changes in their bodies, they try hard to fit in with their peer group. This means slouching a lot while sitting or even while walking. Going to the gym and playing sports, or swimming, cycling or running might not be the 'cool' thing for them to do.

Solution

As for pre-teens, being physically more active, playing sports and exercising more needs to be integrated into the curriculum for teens as well. We need to move on from expecting them to follow what they are told to treating them as adults who can make that decision for themselves. Again, please don't teach subjects just to pass exams, but to actually empower them with knowledge.

Those who are focused on building an academic career usually quit sports and a physically active lifestyle, or are pressurized to do so by 'well-wishers' who encourage them to study hard if they want to get admitted to top colleges.

So, perhaps top colleges and corporates need to get involved in this to encourage young people to become more holistic personalities rather than just being academically driven. Isn't the whole idea that colleges get the best brains and make them even smarter, and top corporates hire the brightest of the bright and grow their businesses even more? How difficult is it then to think long-term and hire people who not only meet current criteria but also have the capability to last longer? That'll only happen if school- and college-going students are physically active along with being academically brilliant.

If the industry rewards physically active lifestyles and exercises along with academics, this age group will be motivated to change its lifestyle. To them, prevention doesn't sell well. This will go a long way in reducing lower back pain.

Adult Years (21–50)

People in this age group are always busy, primarily focused on their career and making money—first for themselves and soon for their young family and elderly parents. To them, even current medical problems like severe back pain aren't of much importance, which sadly they almost always suffer from. But they have no time for themselves. They simply don't get it that if they don't take out some time for themselves now, soon they'll be in a situation where they'll have enough time for themselves but it'll be too late to do anything about their health.

It is a well-established fact that fitness decreases when one spends more than 8 hours sitting in front of the computer, which is almost mandatory in most white-collar jobs in today's world. This leads to back pain. More than half of the working population in cities like Mumbai and

Delhi suffers from back pain of different intensity because of this.

Those who do night shifts, appropriately called 'graveyard shifts', pretty much become typecast at night shift roles and are not offered regular hours. Besides, all the other poor lifestyle habits—going against nature by not sleeping at night, for instance—leads to bigger medical problems. At least one-third of our lives are spent sleeping. There is a good reason for it. Rest and recovery are crucial for us to work at our optimal levels the next day.

Ten years of doing the graveyard shift leads to the brain ageing six extra years. After quitting, it takes another five years to return to your normal health. We need young people to be fit for them to be optimally productive during their peak years. Corporates need to act responsibly to ensure this. Besides outsourcing their jobs to India, it seems the Western world has even outsourced its lifestyle problems and diseases.

Solution

When someone says that they don't have the time to address their pains, it reminds me of the announcements in flights: If you have a small child or an elderly person travelling with you, secure your mask before assisting them with theirs. The same applies in case of those who suffer from back pain but ignore it because of a hectic life dedicated to everyone else.

Sitting for long hours needs to be countered. It is not advisable to have tea and coffee served on your table. There is a reason corporate offices offer that. They want to get the most out of you. Get up and fetch it yourself. Find a reason to get up once every 45 minutes or an hour. Being in any one posture for long isn't good for your back. Keep moving around.

Standing desks are already an option in a few corporate offices. Some even have a workstation at the gym, which I think is a bit too adventurous.

Graveyard shifts are deteriorating the quality of life of today's generation. Drastic steps need to be taken now. The government needs to enforce that corporates have a rehabilitation programme for employees that work the graveyard shift so they can have a longer working career. By regulation, night shifts should be limited to a maximum of three years for any employee. There needs to be mandatory physical fitness assessment every quarter for all employees. Here, the aim should be not to merely test them, but to help them reach their optimal levels of performance.

If you do have a choice, I suggest, even if it means taking a 20–30 per cent cut in your salary, go back to regular day shifts. It'll help you in the long run to address your back pain. You will have a social life again, which is next to impossible for those who work night shifts.

Pregnancy[6]

In today's world, women are focused on their careers and by the time they think they are ready for motherhood, their bodies have already been battered in the rat race. As a result, most women aren't able to cope with the demands of pregnancy and soon enough develop lower back pain, which stays with them even after delivery. Also, babies are more precious now since they are born late and at times using the very strenuous IVF (in-vitro fertilization) process. For this reason, doctors err on the side of caution and suggest the mother-to-be to take care and not indulge in too many physical activities. Parents and parents-in-law suggest the same.

Pregnant women's bodies undergo a lot of emotional, hormonal and musculoskeletal changes. At times, these changes can lead to painful lower back episodes. Almost 60 per cent of pregnant women experience lower back pain at some point. Even though these back pains are by no means life-threatening, they do markedly compromise the quality of life.

Pregnancy is a time of hormonal upheavals. Relaxin is a hormone that leads to loosening ligaments so that the lower back arches further to accommodate the growing foetus. This leads to an increased pressure on the lower back, which soon leads to lower back pain.

A pregnant woman might experience pain in the hips (below the lumbar spine) and the buttocks. This type of pain is usually deep, stabbing, one-sided or covering both sides, continuous or recurrent. The good news is that most of the times this pain subsides after delivery or a few months later. At times, it might radiate down to the thighs and calves. This can be confused with sciatic pain, i.e., pain down the leg because of compression of sciatic nerve in the lower back.

At times, pain is felt in the front of the pelvis, around the pubic area, while turning in the bed or squatting or getting up from a sitting position.

At times, there is pain only on one side of the hip. This pain is associated with movements like changing position while sleeping, getting up, and prolonged standing.

As the uterus increases in size, there is greater weight in front of the abdomen, shifting the body's centre of gravity forward. The body compensates by increasing the arch of the lower back. This, at times, can compress the nerves that branch out at each vertebral level. The fact that abdominal, buttock and pelvic muscles are weak and tight needs to be addressed.

This leads to a domino effect. The chin juts out with a slouching posture, shoulders droop forward, restricting chest expansion, limiting breathing and putting even more pressure on the lower back.

Solution

It is important to understand that pregnancy is not a disease, so continuing optimal physical activity and a daily exercise routine is necessary to ensure better health and a good quality of life. Women, who exercise during pregnancy, can prevent lower back pain, and those who are already suffering from it can markedly reduce it.[7]

Non-specific exercises like walking, swimming, water exercises, stationary cycling and low-impact aerobics are safe (minimal risks if at all) and useful for curing back pain during pregnancy. Exercise and increased physical activity should be done before, during and after pregnancy.

Some women, in their excitement to stay active, might end up participating in sports or activities that can injure them. Please avoid the following during pregnancy: contact sports (ice hockey, boxing, soccer and basketball), activities with a higher risk of falling (downhill skiing, water skiing, surfing, off-road cycling, gymnastics, and horse riding), scuba-diving, skydiving and hot yoga or hot Pilates.

Strengthening abdominal and back muscles is important as well. Simple but specific exercises targeting these areas should be practised regularly.

Case: Bethany Lowe (name changed), thirty-five years old

Ten years ago, a thirty-five-year-old lawyer, practising in London, came to me with lower back pain, which she had been experiencing for fifteen days. There had been an underlying pain for ten years with episodes of severe bouts every three to four months, lasting ten to fifteen days each time. The painful episodes were now getting more frequent, lasting longer, and were more intense. On inquiring further, I learnt that her elder child was ten years old. She then recalled that the very first instance of lower back pain happened in her third trimester of pregnancy when she was pushing a heavy bucket of clothes with her right leg. It immediately caused back and right hip pain.

In spite of having seen a bunch of doctors and therapists, she somehow had never discussed this history before. This led to my colleagues treating the symptoms rather than the cause.

During pregnancy, to accommodate the growing foetus, there is increased laxity of the ligaments of the lower back. If there isn't enough muscle tone and core stability, it leads to the lower back arching forward. Activities that would normally not have bothered her a few months ago, were exposing her to injuries.

On examination, I found out that her right hip was very stiff. The muscles around the right buttock, right lower back and hip were in spasm, not letting the hip move properly and leading to gross muscle imbalance. She had to first unlearn the wrong walking gait she had developed, courtesy this imbalance. This was further aided by corrective exercises that helped her improve her posture and hence her gait. It took four to six weeks to get rid of the lower back pain that she had been living with for a decade.

Case: Neha Yeole, thirty-six years old

Neha Yeole, a thirty-six-year-old mother from Pune shared her story on my running podcast, Move-Mint. She was in

Melbourne for twelve years and got back to India only three years ago. She is a counselling psychologist who deals with patients with chronic physical pain, depression, anxiety, coupled with marital discords, etc.

She suffered from lower back pain soon after having her twins eight years ago. She was advised by an obstetrician in Melbourne to walk and do breathing exercise on a daily basis. Neha religiously did that for a year. After that, she experienced no back pain even after having a very busy personal and professional schedule.

In 2014, Neha met with an accident which resulted in multiple fractures in her left ankle. She was operated upon for the same and had plates and screws put in. After the surgery, she was able to walk. Her doctor was of the opinion that her recovery was a lot quicker because she was up and about a lot sooner than most of the other patients after a similar surgery.

After her own positive experience, Neha now recommends walking to all her patients. She has also started a walking group called 'Walk It Out! Talk It Out', which has over 3,000 members on Facebook and over 250 members on WhatsApp. She says that her patients have come back with success stories after she made them pick up a more physically active lifestyle.

Homemakers

A 2015 study showed that 83 per cent of rural homemakers in Kanpur, in the average age group of 30–70 years, suffered from back pain every year. Half of them had severe disability due to lower back pain and their social lives were severely impacted as a result.[8] Interestingly, the researchers, despite being women, referred to the homemakers as 'non-working'.

Even though, the general notion is that homemakers are unemployed or 'not working', they are working 24x7, without any holiday. They never work for themselves, always for others, and almost always with a bad posture.

The above-mentioned study also showed that lower back pain isn't only an urban phenomenon. Since no one ever asks rural women, or maybe because they are conditioned to never complain and talk about their own problems, back pain is assumed not to be a rural problem.

Solution

Ladies, you need to give yourself priority over everyone and everything else. If you yourself are not fit enough, how will you take care of the whole world? Become more physically active. Taking time out for going out shopping, to the parlour or watching television is important, but equally or more important is taking care of your health. Now, go for an easy walk right now.

Later Working Years (51–65)

Till a couple of decades ago, it was this age group and beyond that would complain of back pain. Surprisingly, now they are in a minority. Most people in this age group have moved their limbs a lot more, not as a recreation but because they didn't have many options. This has given them a solid physical foundation. It is unfortunate to see twenty-to-thirty-year-olds complaining of pain a lot more than their parents.

Solution

Strength training is important but it's important to first simply get moving again. Take time out for yourself. It's not too late; it never is.

Golden Years (over sixty-five years)

I usually find people of this age group fitter than those half their age. It's fascinating sometimes for me to see three generations of a family together in my consultation room, with the oldest being the fittest and the youngest being the most unfit.

Most of them have led a physically active life, but pretty much dedicated to everyone else.

Solution

For those above sixty-five years of age, the plan is to start moving again. Most think walking, running, swimming and cycling are the best exercises but as you age, more than ever, strength training becomes crucial, especially for the back.

The importance of aerobic exercise and strength training was summed up well by Paul Thompson, MD, director of cardiology, Hartford Hospital, in a panel discussion with Dr Steven N. Blair.[9] He said, 'Do aerobic exercise to keep yourself alive, because we've got good evidence on that, but do strength training to keep yourself out of the nursing home.'

Other Stakeholders

Parents

Parents' role is not only limited to conception and giving birth. They decided to bring another human being into this world, so it is their responsibility to be better informed about what is best for the child.

Parents Who are Goal-oriented

In today's hyper-competitive world, parents start planning their children's careers from almost before they are born.

You can't really blame them, especially with the kind of population India is blessed with. Broadly, there are two kinds in this regard.

A majority of them want their children to pursue the traditional, tried and tested academic route. They would have the child privately tutored from an early age so he or she scores well in academics. To them, their children will be defined by the percentage they manage to get in school. Hence they promote a lifestyle where the child is sedentary and doesn't participate in physical activities.

A couple of years ago, I met the principal of one of Delhi's renowned international schools, where at the time my elder son was studying. I was shocked to learn from the boastful principal that she had stopped her daughter's classical dance training in class IX so that the child could focus on studies alone. The principal went on to tell me that her daughter had gone on to do an MBBS from one of the top medical colleges in the country and was now doing post-graduation from another premier institution.

In my opinion, the principal had not only circumscribed her daughter's life but had given the society a doctor who would pass on a faulty philosophy to her patients, one that placed no importance on physical activity. Sadly, the principal didn't realize that she had lost her daughter and created a clone.

What is expected of the students who pass out of that school each year? They will imbibe the same values from the principal, like her daughter did. Apart from other ramifications, the promotion of a sedentary lifestyle will lead to a host of chronic diseases, including back pain.

Parents Who are Sports-oriented

At the other extreme are parents who want to realize their unfulfilled dreams of not having played sports professionally through their children. Maybe their own parents forced them away from sports and towards the traditional academic route, or maybe they didn't make the cut because of an injury or an unfortunate incident. They push their children to achieve in sports what they themselves couldn't. I am completely fine with this if the children have the interest and aptitude for it. Sports shouldn't be thrust on them or on their bodies.

The larger problem remains that these young athletes are not physically fit enough to play sports at a higher level, and are forced into specialization very early in life. This is a perfect recipe for disaster. When, and not if, they do get injured, they will not have enough time to recover and get back to the highest level of performance. Till a child is 10–12 years old, the focus needs to be on overall fitness and multi-sports. This will help them excel in any sport they pick up later and reach their optimal levels of performance without injury.

Young athletes, if they aren't fit enough, might even end up excelling and winning a few medals at the highest level, but will have to suffer the long-term impact of injuries; these can be avoided if they are fitter.

My basic advice to parents of these young sportspersons is that they shouldn't compromise on the health of their daughter or son in the eagerness to create a world champion. I have actually turned away parents who, in an authoritarian mode, are focused on the medal and not the health of their child. Such parents just might win a medal through their child, but in bargain end up giving their child a severe back pain or some other injury that might linger on for a long period of time.

Back pain, by far, is one of the biggest problems unfit sportspersons have to tackle, either because of the injuries they suffered during their playing career or because they had to stop exercising because of other injuries that they incurred while playing.

Case: Sakshi Verma (name changed), fourteen years old

I met the young fourteen-year-old budding golfer in mid-2007. She was suffering from back pain for three months. The pain was so severe now that she wasn't able to carry on with golf. On examining her back, I suspected a stress fracture in her lumbar spine, which was confirmed by an MRI. I advised her to lay off golf for two months, but gave her an exercise programme she could follow during that time.

She was lucky to have a coach (Nonita Qureshi Lall) who didn't take the pain lightly and sought expert advice. She was also a good patient, who followed my recommended exercise programme diligently. She not only got back to playing golf and became India's junior number one, but represented India at the 2010 Asian Games held in Guangzhou, China.

Talent is not enough in sports. At a particular level, it's a given. It's your fitness level that helps you get to a higher level and do justice to your talent. If your fitness doesn't match your talent, you will soon get hurt. This will not only stop you from playing, but cause an injury that will disturb your normal life for a long time.

Pain needs no introduction. It is a reality of life. We all are going to experience it. It's entirely up to us what we make of it and how we handle it. It is suffering that is optional. Giving up on pain is not an option that you have. You need to be in control.

As my mentor in musculoskeletal medicine, Dr Roderic Macdonald said: 'Pain is only a messenger. You appreciate it and respect it. But then you need to move on.' That's what you need to do too.

Solution: Buddha (or Wise) Parents

In a child's life, a parent's role is far greater than anyone else's—including teachers. There is no right or wrong in parenting, but at all times the parents must put the child at the centre of all their decisions. Once a parent does that, the future approach becomes a lot clearer.

'Small factors' come into play from the time a child is born. Parents become very protective of their children, obviously with good intentions of keeping them out of trouble, but it backfires too. Parents stop them from making that extra effort, hence the child's mind or body is not able to adapt optimally to the demands of the real world. Parents need to encourage the children to move and play so that they can be independent.

The child is impressionable and picks up whatever the parents do. Parents being physically fit and leading a healthy lifestyle will make a big difference to the child. Children pick up actions more than what is preached to them.

Children whose mothers are highly educated are more likely to be in excellent or very good health, irrespective of the household. Also, if mothers are in good to excellent health, their children are more likely to have good health themselves. On the other hand, children whose parents have specific health problems are more likely to have the same health problems.[10] Parental exercise may influence their children's participation in extracurricular sports and cardiorespiratory fitness levels.[11]

This possibly is because educated parents are more aware of benefits of physical activity and a healthy lifestyle.

It is possibly also because they tend to have better priorities in life rather than just making more money. Hence parents, not doctors, are the primary gatekeepers of their children's health.

Most parents follow the do-as-I-say-not-as-I-do philosophy. We all know that doesn't really work. It has repeatedly been shown that more than movie and sports celebrities, youngsters look up to their own parents as role models. This is why we all need to be more aware of what we do. You need to be a worthy role model as a parent. If you are the one always seated in front of the idiot box, you've got a serious problem. Even worse is if your favourite asana is the Vishnu pose, i.e., you are almost always lying down while watching the television or reading the newspaper. That's exactly what your kids would do too.

In today's fast-paced world, adults are always on their smartphones and have no time for their children. Children aspire to a similar lifestyle with gadgets. For you the easiest way to cater to your child's needs from as early as two to three years of age is to give them a smartphone or a tablet so that it keeps them occupied and they don't bother you. In doing so, you have created a long-term problem for your kids. You have messed them up for life both psychologically and physically.

A couple of decades ago, children used to be running all over the house and the courtyard and wouldn't even sit down to watch television. That's what humans were supposed to do. Move. Not just sit in front of the idiot box. Parents now get them gadgets not because it is a necessity but because they don't have time to entertain their children.

I often see parents coming to the clinic, worried that their ten- or eleven-year-old child has severe back pain; something even they don't have yet. Just look back. Thank your own parents and your upbringing. It's now time to pass it on to your kids. Sometimes they are too old to listen to you any more. The good news is, it's never too late. Make the change now. Lead by example. Children will pick it up soon enough. They always look up to you, even if they can't find the right words to describe it.

It's all very well to plan their careers, but first remember that they are your responsibility. Not just future moneymaking machines or trophies that you can only be proud of their accomplishments. Whether it is academic, sports or both that you want them to excel in, think about long-term investment. If they are healthy, they will be able to achieve much more.

By doing so, you are saving them from a lifetime of back pain issues. Keep them active throughout their lives. By being a 'Buddha parent' and following the Buddha's middle path approach in parenting, you'll help them and yourself at the same time.

Teachers

Teachers aren't immune to back pain. Long drives to school, standing and then sitting for extended periods of time, coupled with a hectic but physically inactive life, puts you at a high risk of severe back pain. If you are teaching junior classes, bending down or sitting on small chairs puts more pressure on your lower back and aggravates the problem.

Even if you look at it very selfishly, wouldn't it be fun to look and feel a couple of decades younger? The changes you make in your students could simply be a by-product of becoming healthier yourself.

Like parents, what teachers say or do impacts children for life. Unfortunately, they aren't appreciated enough for their efforts. Without the active support of teachers, no problem can be addressed, even that of back pain. Again, you need to lead by example rather than just preaching anything. There will be a lot more conviction in your statements if you have experienced the benefits yourself. Don't you hate it when you consult a doctor who is as spherical as planet earth!

It's not only the physical education or sports teacher who should be thinking about the fitness and health of students. Students are very impressionable till the age of 11–12. After that, it becomes harder to get through to them. Hence these foundation years are crucial. All teachers should make an effort to stay active themselves and lead a healthy lifestyle. Physical activity, exercises and sports can easily be integrated with any subject that you teach. Once you are able to address the unasked questions of the ever-inquisitive young students, you've got yourself converts for life.

Solution

It becomes the job of enthusiastic, physically active teachers, not necessarily sports fanatics, to spread the attitude and behaviour that prioritize these values to every other teacher on campus. Don't wait for the school authorities to take the initiative. They'll follow once you get started.

Below are some questions that you need to respond to:

a) Do you have occasional neck, middle or lower back or knee pain? Or is it more severe?
b) Do you currently suffer from any chronic diseases?
c) Do you get breathless from climbing a single or a couple of flights of stairs?
d) Can you not do a brisk walk for even a kilometre?
e) Are you sleeping less than 7 to 8 hours a day?

f) Are you sitting (including travel) for more than 6 hours a day?
g) Do you miss breakfast or have a very light one?

If you answered 'yes' to any of the above questions, you are a good candidate to start moving a little bit more and making healthier lifestyle choices, including better eating habits. Wouldn't it be wonderful if you could address your poor health and take steps to change it? Here are some ideas about how you can do this:

a) Weekly teachers' meet: This does not even need external experts. Teachers from different departments and backgrounds could come together and discuss the problems at hand and chart out a plan. You don't need extra time for this. Do it during lunch. Spare 15 to 30 minutes a week for this.
b) Primary catalyst: Initially, the teachers who are fitness enthusiasts could talk for 5 minutes about what clicks for them and what lifestyle changes have helped them in their lives.
c) Motivator of the week: Soon enough, you can have teachers who are new to the programme to share their challenges and how baby steps have helped them overcome their hesitancy to get moving. Other teachers will relate better to their stories and experiences since now it's one of them who is talking about making basic changes.
d) Short exercises: Start each class by asking students to rotate their shoulders up and down, move them back and forth, ten to fifteen times. End the same way.
e) Standing classes: Have two classes daily where you and the students are standing throughout. Tell the students

that it's not a punishment. They are just giving you company. It's fine if they lean against their desks. At least you'll get them and yourself off your backsides.

f) Free classes in a playground: If the subject teacher is absent, and you are only there as a replacement, make it a point to take the students out to an open area or, even better, to a playground. You could make them do rounds of the ground. The students will have fun and get some exercise. It's good for you too.

g) Ten-minute alarms: Ten minutes into your lesson or period, ask all the students to get up from their chairs and raise their arms and try and touch the ceiling. Hold that for 4 seconds and bring them back down again. Do five repetitions. You need to lead this activity.

h) Lighter bags: Randomly inspect bags of students just to check how heavy they are. Encourage them to lighten their bags.

i) Shoes off: For a period or two a day, ask the students to knock off their shoes. It surprisingly calms down the back and leg muscles.

The above are good ways to get you to be more active. Once you've done this for a couple of months, you can pick activities and exercises mentioned earlier.

Soon you'll be enjoying a new 'you'. Congratulate yourself for beginning your silent movement against a lifetime of back pain.

Doctors

As Beneficence's quote goes, *Salus aegroti suprema lex*, i.e., a practitioner should act in the best interest of the patient. Doctors are considered custodians of the healthcare industry.

That's why being a doctor is being in a noble profession. We all need to start playing a far more important role. Let's all get our patients moving more.

The March 2011 issue of the *British Journal of Sports Medicine* (*BJSM*), a premiere sports medicine journal, had a review of *Physical Activity in the Prevention and Treatment of Disease*, a groundbreaking book by the Professional Associations for Physical Activity (Sweden). *BJSM* suggested that every doctor's consultation room should have a copy of the free PDF and it had to be used twenty to thirty times daily.

Dr Anurag Mishra, a doctor friend, agrees. He recently confessed, 'I think "fitness" is one of those words whose meaning you realize only if you get it, even losing it may not help you realize what it is.' Anurag is really making an effort. After being a slob and not exercising for many years, he can now run/walk for 20 km at a stretch.

We doctors simply don't know about fitness or exercise till we ourselves make an effort. You need to be a student again to appreciate their full benefit rather than just rubbishing it or saying you know it all without knowing any better, simply because as a doctor you are under the pressure of knowing everything and anything.

Clinicians have an ethical obligation to prescribe physical activity, but then what is stopping them? What are the barriers?

During undergraduate medical studies, since the focus is on passing examinations, no one thinks much about exercise, fitness or lifestyle changes that all textbooks mention as the primary approach to address chronic diseases. Even our teachers barely spend any time on this. We end up not knowing enough about the importance of exercise and physical activities. How then do we even have the right to give advice on the same to anyone else? But we do, without knowing enough ourselves.

When we get to our speciality training, we are too narrowly focused on it. By now it's too late to know anything about something so fundamental. Even doctors specializing in relevant fields on lower back pain, such as orthopaedics, rheumatology, neurology, anaesthesiology and internal medicine, just don't have the time to expand the horizons of their knowledge and look beyond their topic.

When we start practising medicine, we again become too busy and have no time to understand the basics any more. Also by now, we are rooted in the foundation of our training, which is purely based on catering to illness, and not well-being. The idea is to make people less ill. We don't know what the human body is capable of, but we are aware of what the limitations of the human body are. By now, we either don't advise exercise and increased physical activity, or if we do, almost always, it is the wrong advice.

I urge fellow doctors to stop prescribing complete bed rest, which is not considered the right thing to do any more. Please stop prescribing MRIs for back pain at the drop of a hat. Electrotherapeutic modalities used by physiotherapists have no role in curing chronic back pain.

When it comes to our personal lives, we doctors aren't actually doing any better. Even if we happen to have the correct knowledge on the subject of exercise and increased physical activity, we simply are so busy making a career and improving our bank balance that we forget even about our own selves. Soon enough, the shape of our bodies changes to either cylindrical or spherical. Now, even if we want to advise our patients to be physically active throughout the day and exercise regularly, we don't have much credibility. Since we haven't been able to lead a healthy lifestyle ourselves, there is no conviction in our advice either.

Since we have no time for our families, courtesy our busy schedule, we buy them expensive gifts and gadgets to keep them occupied. Soon enough, they are hooked on to these and do not care when you start talking about a healthy lifestyle. You need to lead by example, not preach something that is alien to you.

Solution

There is only one way to bring about a change in your lives as doctors and to your patients', and that is to start exercising. A healthy doctor automatically inspires patients to have healthy lifestyles, thereby reducing incidences of back pain.

As a medical community, we need to encourage each other to choose healthy lifestyles for life. When we meet during medical conferences, I suggest we spend time discussing our health problems. We should follow it up with a section dedicated to different exercises and other physical activities. It's important for all chronic diseases, including cancer, not just back pain.

There is already a move to have exercise and increased physical activity named as an important component in medical schools in the UK. The same needs to happen in India too. It's difficult to make things happen once students are out of their medical schools.

Once you become an ideal doctor, my purpose is solved. Your patients will automatically do what you do. A lot more patients will start taking their lower back pains a lot more positively. They'll be open to conservative pain management.

You'll have to come down to their level to make a change at the grass-roots level.

What Causes Back Pain

School Bags

A UK-based charity, BackCare's study suggests that 80 per cent of kids who carry as little load as one-fifth (20 per cent) of their body weight, are really taxing their bodies. Studies have shown that even carrying more than ten per cent of your body weight can cause spinal damage. This is pretty much happening from the moment children start going to school. This is the beginning of long-term damages. Dr Peter Skew, an Essex-based expert of musculoskeletal medicine and (former) vice-president of BackCare (from whom I took over the position as in-house doctor at Kieser Training, London) says, 'We are seeing increasing numbers of young adults coming for treatment in relation to back trouble and this can often be traced back to carrying heavy bags to school.

'Children's skeletons are still developing, and having a heavy bag slung over one shoulder can exert unnatural force on the spine . . . rather like exercising only one side of your body in the gym, you quickly get unilateral muscle loading, which can cause the small muscles in the back to tighten and compress the spine.'

You would think that institutions would pay attention to literally the backbone of tomorrow's leaders. These studies have been reported in national newspapers across the globe, but I haven't seen any institution taking any concrete actions.

To make matters worse, in schools today, sport is not a priority, only academics is. I see enough people in their early twenties with severe back pain. Other than the heavy bags, growing number of schools give homework that is to be done on computers and then leisure time is spent lazing around in front of the TV, eating junk food.

Chairs and Sitting

Sitting is called the new smoking. It is because physical inactivity is the fourth largest killer. We humans simply weren't made to be stationary. We were made to move.

It was only 500 years ago that the masses started using chairs, up until then chest of drawers, benches and stools were used in everyday living. With the Industrial Revolution a mere 260 years ago, human beings took the sedentary lifestyle to a whole new level. Computers have only been around for the last fifty years, at a mass scale for less than half that time, but they have changed things way too quickly. In addition to that, the way we travel (cars) and eat (fast food) today has changed our lives for the worse. Tablets and smartphones came into being at the beginning of this millennium and have done their bit to add to our sedentary lifestyles.

Most of us prefer using chairs with wheels, where our feet are not grounded and we are not stable. Sitting on a chair and at a computer is a deadly combination. Whether barefoot or not, there is a desperate need for human beings to feel the ground again.

Driving a Car

Improper seat height and angle while driving can cause unnecessary tension in the neck, upper, middle or lower back.

Men usually have their seats further back and women have them too low. Even if your car doesn't address seat height, adjust it by keeping a support below. If your seat is too reclined, you will slouch and jut your head out to make out where the front of the car is. It's always better to have the car seat higher so your head and back are supported. If your lower back is still uncomfortable, place a rolled-up towel there according to your comfort level. Your arms should be bent a little at the elbows, for which your steering wheel needs to be closer to you.

Case: Rajesh Chopra (name changed), thirty-eight years old

A businessman from Delhi, who has his export factory in Gurgaon, was experiencing lower back pain and pain down the left leg for seven to eight months. He is an active fitness enthusiast who is not into sports but goes to the gymnasium on a regular basis. Gym activity could refer to any permutation or combination of doing strength training on the machines or floor, group classes (stretches, yoga, Pilates, etc.) or cardiovascular exercises. He mainly focuses on group classes and not on strength training.

He is very careful not to lift any heavy boxes at work. His workstation is as good as it possibly can be. He limits his phone and computer usage. He is up and about on his feet every hour or so. Basically, he had been taking good care of himself. On asking about the changes in his life at the time the pain began, he remembered that about nine months ago he purchased a second hand, three-year-old, high-end SUV (sports utility vehicle) that he drove for 3 to 4 hours a day. He admitted that the clutch of the SUV was a bit tight. In a city like Delhi, you need to use the clutch a lot more than an accelerator while driving.

Besides coming up with immediate pain relief solution and giving him corrective exercises, which is never difficult for people who are already into fitness, I was able to convince him to sell off his SUV and buy an automatic car in the same budget. He has been driving the same distances and there is no pain any more.

Driving a Bus

I use this topic to showcase that sometimes we just assume that since something is so obvious that it'll just make sense to people and it'll be implemented.

The classical London double-decker bus study[12] done in 1949 was the first that showed the impact of modern sedentary lifestyle on cardiovascular disease. It involved 31,000 London transport workers and compared the sedentary lives of drivers with that of the active life of conductors. Both had eight-hour shifts, six days a week. While the bus drivers sat all day, the conductors ran up and down the two levels of the bus. It was found that the drivers were suffering from cardiovascular diseases and dying sooner than the conductors. Had the researchers looked for it, the same would have been the case for back pain. Just that back pain wouldn't have killed them but would have made their lives miserable.

You would have thought that London would have promoted active lifestyle by carrying on with the old-style, rear-open buses where conductors would run up and down the two floors. What they actually did in 2006 was replace them by buses with automatic doors which didn't need any conductors.

A 2012 Kolkata study[13], involving 160 male bus drivers in a public sector transport company, observed that all of them suffered with lower back pain. The bus drivers did eight- to ten-hour shifts daily for six days a week. Pain restricted their social and professional life. Bus drivers across the country are highly stressed, both physically and psychologically, due to the hazardous working conditions, which affects their health and overall work performance in the long run.

Solution

As much as it would seem that no change is expected in your situation if the employers aren't interested in doing anything about it, you have to be in control, it is your body. There is always a solution, but only if you look for it.

Sitting stationary in any one position for the whole day is not good for you.

Stressed-out bus drivers in all Indian cities suffer from back pain. Since we know that long sitting isn't good for the back, we need to address that. It needs to come out as a policy from the government.

The work environment needs to be better, helping the employees become fitter. One way of achieving this is by providing adequate number of breaks for the bus drivers. Policies need to be put into place to ensure that the number of hours is restricted as is done in the case of pilots and flying crews with rest days built into the schedule. For the same reason, in cricket, fast bowlers are allowed to bowl a fixed number of spells in a day.

Gadgets: Computers, Laptops, Tablets, Smartphones

A recent study[14] looked at the top young video gamers whose reaction times would put fighter pilots to shame. One leading gamer in his twenties appeared to be slim and healthy with a physique not dissimilar to an endurance athlete, but had the lung function and aerobic fitness of a sixty-year-old chain-smoker. So, just body size and obesity as a scale to measure fitness may not really be accurate. Physical activity is very important. Sitting in front of computers for long hours is also messing up the sitting posture and leading major muscle imbalances. Strength training on a regular basis, at least three times a week, plays an important role to improve the posture.

Too much typing on flat electronic surfaces will make you push your shoulders further back, in effect causing tension in the neck and upper back. Excessive reading on these devices can also lead to poor posture—rounded shoulders, stiff upper back and increased pressure on the lower back. This can cause neck pain and middle and lower back pain.

Solution

Don't worry if your employers aren't interested in doing anything about it, you have to be in control—it is your body. There is always a solution, but only if you look for it.

Sitting stationary in any one position for the whole day is not good for you. You were made to move, you need to keep moving. Don't keep sitting at your workstation or in a meeting for more than 45 minutes. Find a reason to get up—to fetch a glass of water or go to the washroom. Whatever it might be, I want you to move.

Shoes

We spend more than half our lives wearing shoes (or some sort of footwear). Why is it then that we don't pay enough attention to ensure the shoes are comfortable? If the footwear doesn't feel right, it's only making things worse for you.

Minimalist and barefoot running has become popular, courtesy the book with a cult following, *Born to Run*. However, barefoot or minimalist running isn't magical. Shoes, or the lack of them, are not going to improve your running technique. Only if the shoes are appropriate for you do they temporarily and artificially help you correct your flat foot or overpronation of feet, i.e., excess rolling in of the foot when you walk, because of poor arches of the feet. Shoes work like bumpers of a car. The cushioning helps in reducing the impact on the feet, knees and the back. You wouldn't want to drive a Mercedes without the bumpers. Same goes for the body.

Solution

As a rule of thumb, leather-soled heels are not good for you. Also, size is an important aspect. Your sports shoes need to be a size bigger than your formal shoes. Brand loyalty can also lead to problems.

For long-term and permanent improvement of walking and running technique, your muscle imbalances need to be corrected. Once you do that, even the most basic shoes will work for you. But till then, look for a shoe that addresses your weak foot arches.

In the medical community, for a while now, shoe insoles (orthotics) have been thought to play a very important role in preventing and treating lower back pain, but the most recent studies[15] looking at more than 30,000 people with back pain found that shoe insoles don't play a significant enough role in preventing an episode of lower back pain.

Smoking[16]

Smoking has an effect on lower back pain. Smokers are three times more likely to develop lower back pain than non-smokers. The nicotine in cigarettes is known to cause thickening of the walls in our blood vessels, such as arteries. This also extends to the blood vessels that circulate the flow of blood to the muscle groups that protect the vertebrae, nerves and, to a lesser extent, the disc.

Progressive narrowing of blood vessels results in loss of circulation of protective blood cells, oxygen and nutrients, and delay in removal of waste products. Blood supply, healing and recovery are slower and less efficient. The potential for muscle injury and damage is higher for smokers.

The Big Thick Wallet in the Back Pocket

Men who put wallets in their back pockets throw the whole spine completely out of alignment. Eyes do a good job of working like a spirit level. If your pelvis is higher on one side because of the wallet in the back pocket, rest of the spine will turn and twist a bit (scoliosis) to keep the eyes and head straight. Soon enough this adapted posture becomes a habit and contributes to headache, neck pain and lower back pain.

Directly, the wallet in the back pocket compresses the piriformis muscle, which lies directly over the sciatic nerve. This can easily irritate the sciatic nerve. This causes pain in the buttocks and one might also experience a sharp pain going down the leg. This is called sciatica.

Solution

A simple way to avoid this is to keep your wallet in the front pocket of your trousers or your jacket pocket. Luckily,

50 per cent of the population (women) doesn't do that. Yet, they have a different problem—the handbag!

Women's Handbags

Women make up for it by carrying handbags. This causes malalignment of the spine as they either lower or raise the shoulder on which the bag in slung across. This again leads to permanent changes in the posture, soon enough leading to back pain.

Solution

The best way to cater to this is to keep the handbag as light as possible and keep switching hands rather than holding it in one hand alone.

Laptop Bags

This again causes an imbalance in your spine. The straps also dig into your upper back muscles and trigger pain.

Solution

Always have your laptop bags on both the shoulders and don't have the straps too low. It's often seen that the youth have their laptop bags very low, at times the bag is as low as the buttock. This puts pressure on the upper and the lower back. This further leads to poor posture, and in due course causes back pain.

Ponytails

If hair is pulled back too tight, it can start causing tension first in your head and then in your neck muscles. Before you know, your head is jutting out and you have a slouched posture.

Solution

It's best not to tie your hair too tight. Sometimes even after the trigger is removed, pain continues.

Wrong-sized Bra

It might come as a surprise to most women, but wearing wrong-sized bras can lead to headache and pain in the back, neck and shoulders. Majority of women don't bother to get the right-sized bras. Some end up wearing the wrong size on purpose, either a size too big or too small, depending on how they want to make their cleavage and breasts appear.

Straps of smaller bras can dig into the shoulders and compress nerves, muscles and blood vessels. On the other hand, a bra that is too big can lead to postural problems like rounded shoulders and slouched back. If the straps are too tight, they restrict chest expansion during breathing. One needs to understand that the band that goes around the chest is far more important than the shoulder straps.

Solution

Today all good brands that sell lingerie do proper fitting for bras. Every six months, it is important that women get themselves fitted properly and know their correct bra size that is recommended by the experts there. This simple but very important tip could address a lot of aches and pains. It's important to wear sports bras while exercising as breasts tend to move.

Where Back Pain Is Caused

Most people complain of the environment since they know it can't change much. The onus lies on you. Start making micro changes and macro will soon happen. We all need to lead by example.

Educational Institutions: Schools and Colleges

Crèches, preschools, schools and colleges play a very vital role in children's lives. We are made to believe that these institutions are building a sound foundation for our next generation. In my opinion, as far as physical fitness and back pain go, they are messing up whatever is left of the sound foundation, which we were born with anyway.

It doesn't help if the youth today have a very sound and sharp brain if it resides in an unhealthy body. It doesn't take a degree to understand that. Maybe it's better not to have degrees to understand this. As many as half the students in middle and senior schools suffer from back pain. Till a couple of decades ago, back pain was considered a problem that only senior citizens faced.

Playgrounds are disappearing from school campuses, and so are the sports education classes. Instead, school bags are getting heavier and heavier. Even kids less than ten years of age carry bags as heavy as themselves.

The Problem: Aping the West

Let's learn from our own past by delving deeper into the Ramayana and the Mahabharata era. During those days the gurukuls focused on giving equal importance to body, mind and soul. Pupils were considered unworthy if they didn't pay enough attention in all three, and that too in an integrated manner.

Our age-old yoga in its modern avatar refers to a set of stretching exercises and occasionally breathing exercises as well. It might surprise you, but that only comprises 5–10 per cent of what yoga is supposed to be. Some of you might be aware but yoga is more than just asanas and pranayama—it also includes *yama*, *niyama*, *pratyahara*, *dharana*, dhyana and samadhi. Yoga, in its true sense, is not only about a set of stretching and breathing exercises alone. It's a way of life.

In today's modern society, because of the tough competition, entry requirements to get into top institutions are so rigorous that at times even perfect scores aren't enough to guarantee admission. Parents get their children into this rat race so early that there is no time for childhood. Schools start catering to this need from the very beginning. We doctors add to the confusion by not giving very sound advice whether for medicines, physical activity or food. We prescribe antibiotics and sugary foods like biscuits very early on in life for short-term gains, ignoring long-term repercussions completely.

We all forget that we are dealing with human beings. We are just busy creating more of the same, soulless robots. In this whole process, we don't realize that the current system, by focusing on academics alone, only manages to make children reach at best one-third of body–mind–soul approach followed a few millenniums ago.

Somehow, down the ages, super-specialities have overtaken, forgetting the very basics. It's now all about return on investment and instant gratification. If the foundation isn't very strong, how do we expect to build all those mega dreams on them? Sooner than later, it'll all come tumbling down. As a matter of fact, this is what is happening all around us.

Today's youth is very emotionally and physically fragile, the other two pillars of education that even top institutions aren't able to address. Children in middle and high school, leave alone college-going youth, are already having mental breakdowns and are going into depression. It comes naturally to them from a very early age to figure out a smartphone or a tablet, but they struggle to climb a flight of stairs or walk a kilometre or even sit by themselves for a moment without having suicidal thoughts. This generation's reaction time might be as good as a top fighter pilot but they physically and emotionally are weaker than people four to five decades older than them. Even if they do live long enough courtesy all the advancements in medical technology, their quality of life will be far worse. What good is all that knowledge if it's going to fail this current generation when they are supposed to be in their prime of professional productivity? A thought that somehow doesn't bother the top educationists today!

Solution: Start from the Kids

When it comes to authorities in educational institutions, I am somehow very wary as I have often been told, 'We've been doing it for so long, what can you tell us.' Such inflated egos need to be punctured if we are looking at any change. If we are interested in making a difference, we need to let go of the ego and think beyond ourselves.

Sports and physical activities can no longer be treated as extra-curricular. Sports need to be incorporated into all the subjects being taught in school so that all students are repeatedly exposed to it.

Parents and teachers, whom the children look up to as role models, need to lead by example.

There should be grades for sports and fitness. Sports should carry equal weightage as other subjects. The moment grades get impacted by not following a healthy lifestyle, children will make the right choices.

There is a need to have parents' forums started by doctors and teachers. Several studies have shown that community living and having a group of friends who think alike helps bring about a change in mindsets. There is a need to create a forum where like-minded parents interact with others and encourage each other to follow good practices.

Teachers should be given an incentive to lead a better lifestyle and in coming years it should be a prerequisite to get the job as a teacher.

As much as I believe in multimode approaches to address a problem as complex and serious as this, we need to start somewhere. Children are the seeds of the society, the future. We need to start from them. Children under the age of twelve years form a very substantial part (25 per cent of the Indian population today). They are also very mouldable till that age. As Mahatma Gandhi said, 'Be the change that you wish to see in the world.' Parents, teachers and doctors, the three sets of people whom children interact most with, need to lead by example. It's a very fundamental three-pronged approach for all of us based on an age-old adage: I hear and I forget, I see and I remember, I do and I understand.

The thing to remember is that incentives drive behaviour. We might complain that a large majority of teachers in India are not setting a good example as they are not physically active. There simply is no incentive to be any different. Teachers see no benefit in following healthy lifestyles or to make the children fitter.

The benefits are of course there, but they may not be as tangible in the shorter term. This is where leadership plays a big role—we can make one or two changes and design incentives to drive the right behaviours.

Healthcare Industry

We need to make our healthcare industry fitter and healthier and lead by example. Enough has been covered about it throughout the chapter, so I would not delve deeper into this here. Just a note though, the current healthcare system, even in its best avatar, is a passive one. Unless you, the one with aches and pains, take responsibility for your own self and do something about it, nothing will change.

Medical students and practising doctors need to be trained in exercise medicine and its role in tackling chronic diseases. Doctors need to be encouraged to pick up sports and exercises. This way, they will sound more convincing when they talk about it.

Make each medical interaction count by asking, assessing and prescribing exercise and increased physical activity during each consultation. Obstetricians, gynaecologists and paediatricians need to lead by example. It makes a lot more sense to preach a healthy lifestyle if they practise that good lifestyle themselves. Doctors should encourage people to become a lot more physically active, improve eating habits, which primarily means cutting down on sugar and sweet beverages, and take out 15 to 30 minutes to unwind every day. Medical associations and councils need to encourage this practice by giving benefits to fitter doctors. Over time, it becomes a prerequisite for doctors to lead a healthy lifestyle.

Government

The elected government should be interested in long-term gains for the society but most candidates only want to impress their vote banks so they can get re-elected.

Political and industry leaders are going on and on about India having the second largest workforce in the world, next only to China, when it is actually the largest *unfit* workforce. If India intends to compete with upcoming economies, it needs to invest in its future, that is the health of its youth. They should take some cues from our very own Mahatma Gandhi who didn't have Twitter, Facebook and other social media to spread his word, so he walked pretty much all over India. Our leaders need to set an example for the youth to follow.

I will give you an example. I was invited to write a white paper for a new sports university in Delhi. My only condition for working on the project was to be allowed to think outside the box. The impact of a project like this can be seen in the population earliest in five years, but a far bigger difference will be discernible in a decade. I soon realized the government was keener on short-term gains as it would be of no use to them if the results came after their current term was over.

The learning in this is that it's a matter of our health. It is feasible not to leave it to others to solve it for you and then blame them for not meeting your expectations. You are your own responsibility. Take everything you get from others as a bonus. Stop complaining about poor infrastructure if you can't take care of that one infrastructure that you are fully responsible for, which is your own body. Start moving from today. Soon enough, even the worst infrastructure will seem brilliant.

Solution

There is a need to look at urban designing to encourage active transport. Active transport is the most practical and sustainable way to increase physical activity on a daily basis. More than encouragement and motivation, ease of doing activities is important.

The government needs to develop safe pavements and cycling paths that are well integrated with public transport.

The society needs to come together to promote walking, cycling and usage of public transport.

Mass media and social media needs to be used to spread the awareness and change social norms on physical activity. Social media needs to be used by schools, colleges, corporates and the public sector to promote a more active lifestyle.

If it takes a Modi for Indians to understand that cleanliness and yoga are good, let's also have him and other thought leaders show the way in this as well. Let's all lead by example.

Your Job

Globally lower back pain[17] is the leading, and neck pain[18] is the fourth leading cause of global disability among all medical conditions. Almost one out of every ten people in the world suffers from lower back pain. It is no different in India, whether rural or urban, men or women, young or old. Back pain directly or indirectly leads to major losses to the corporate world, not only in the form of medical expenses but loss of working days and reduced efficiency.

By their late twenties or early thirties, because of sitting for an immense amount of time on a chair in front of a computer screen, a lot of people not only have a bad back but also poor overall health. Both extremes—sedentary and physically demanding jobs—are not good. Repeatedly lifting, pulling, or anything that twists the spine may contribute to back pain.

Solution: Facility Management (FM) Professionals Take a Proactive Role

Earlier I was of the opinion that most corporate companies would rather lose the employee with aches and pains than try to fix the problem. It works in their favour (it's less hard work and cheaper) to get new employees. Hence, they ignore the mega problem. You, as an employee, have added to this attitude because of switching jobs every two months.

On 1 July 2016, I was invited as the keynote speaker by Knowledge Hour, Facility Management Zone, North India Chapter to share my insights on 'Healthy Lifestyle, Workplace Ergonomics and Its Relevance in Today's Corporate World'. This is a quarterly meeting of the senior facilities management professionals who are members of the knowledge-based, pan-India initiative, FM Zone. These get-togethers help all FM colleagues to connect better, share knowledge, share experiences and to establish professional relationships within the fraternity.

This changed my opinion of the corporate world. Over 300 facility managers gathered together on a rainy evening. In spite of the heavy traffic and the bad weather, they were there to improve the working conditions of the employees in their facilities. They all were genuinely interested in everything I had to say even though my turn to speak came only at 9 p.m. We need to use such platforms to share ideas and to get support.

Solution: Ergonomic Bodies

Even though there is an emphasis on workstations with ergonomic furniture, it is important that we first focus on making our bodies ergonomic. In my opinion, the expensive ergonomic chairs only benefit the bank accounts of companies manufacturing and selling them. Even a simple stool works perfectly well, if we know how to use our body appropriately.

A study[19] that looked at over a million people, showed that it takes a brisk walk of 60 to 75 minutes to reverse the damage all day sitting does. No amount of ergonomic furniture can replace that.

Solution: Corporate Employee Responsibility—Time to Walk the Talk

As mentioned earlier, besides breast cancer, heart attacks, obesity and stroke, ten years of graveyard (night and midnight) shifts leads to six extra years ageing of the brain. After quitting, it takes another five years to return to normal. We need our youth to be fit for longer, for them to be optimally productive during their peak years. Corporates need to be held responsible for this.

The government needs to enforce the corporates to have a rehabilitation programme for such employees so that they can have a long working career.

By regulation, night shifts should be limited to three years for any employee. There needs to be mandatory physical fitness assessment every quarter for all employees.

Insurance Companies

I would have thought that insurance companies would rather have physically active people but somehow they don't seem very keen. It is probably because of lack of a long-term vision or not thinking beyond their own individual selves.

Some insurers and third-party payers have little incentive to reduce disability. This is sad but true. The 'what's-in-it-for-me' attitude is a problem. On top of that, they aren't much interested in your well-being, because their own volume of business or profit margin depends on both the volume of cases and duration of disability (i.e., total payouts).

Solution

The business model for insurance companies should be to have as many healthy people insured by them and also to keep all who are insured as healthy as possible. Why should any insurance company want to pay for expensive surgeries? These insurance companies need to make an image in the public domain that they care for their clients' health. They should sponsor events that promote activities like walking, running, etc.

Sports and Back Pain

Sports, exercise and physical activities like running, lawn tennis, squash, cricket (especially fast bowling), basketball, horse riding, football, gym exercises, etc., if done without good fitness levels or done with poor technique, have a far higher chance of leading to back pain.

Most people pick up sports, exercises and increased physical activities to stay fit, but soon end up getting injuries, with back and knee being the commonest area affected. As ironical as it may seem, people who stay inactive have underlying injuries, but since they don't move, it seems to them that they don't have the injuries that the physically active people do.

For the folks on a mission, please stay on track, you are on the right one. Just keep in mind that to prevent and even manage back pain while doing these activities, you have to have both basic fitness and activity-specific fitness. You have to first answer a question for yourself: Are you fit enough to play your chosen sport?[20] Weird question, since you picked sports and exercises to get fit in the first place.

Underperformance and repeatedly getting injured are common signs of not being fit at a fundamental level. This is relevant to both elite professionals and amateur sportspersons. Most enthusiasts love their sport and just want to get on with it without doing the 'boring' warm-up, cool-down, stretching or strengthening. Even if they end up in a gym, they will do the jazzy stuff—not what they should, because they don't know any better.

Amongst those who are able to make the cut and become professional sportspersons, talent seems to be overrated. We Indians seem to be experts at producing junior world champs who are non-existent by the time they are in the senior category. This is because they have either got injured or have not been able to keep up with the physical fitness levels of international players. However, the truth is that at the highest level of the game (any game) talent is taken for granted—else they wouldn't have made the cut. What differentiates the men from the boys, or the women from the girls, is their physical fitness level.

If someone is only playing sports to stay active and for holistic development, they need to start with general fitness. They need to work on three broad areas—strengthening, stretching and cardiovascular workouts, all of which are required for general well-being and are common to all sports.

Sports like running, golf, lawn tennis, squash, cricket (fast bowlers), football, basketball, badminton, etc., expose you to more injuries like back and neck pain.

Most golf players, who do strength training, make the mistake of focusing on 'beach muscles' or 'Salman muscles', i.e., biceps, pectorals, a six-pack and so on, without focusing on the upper back, the lower back or legs. A pioneer in golf-specific injuries, Ramsay McMaster used to call them the 'deadly sins of golf', because working solely on these muscles leads to major muscle imbalances. It's a recipe for disaster.

They need to focus on general overall body fitness and sports specific exercises especially to strengthen the lower back muscles and stretch the ilio-psoas (deep hip and inner thigh muscles) in this case. Else, they will repeatedly keep getting hurt, their standard of playing won't seem to improve, and they won't seem all that keen on it as a career either.

Golf[21] has been considered an older person's sport and many mistakenly believe that you don't need a high level of fitness in order to play it. Yet, top golfers prove that you need to be as athletic for golf as for any other sport.

Technique plays an important role as well. In a sport such as golf, incorrect technique can lead to back pain, which is the primary reason for back injuries among both amateurs and professionals.

The golf swing is not a natural movement and is not very back-friendly, even if the best techniques are employed. Poor technique and repetition, more than the swing itself, are the main reasons for back pain in golf players. There is compression and excessive torsion of the spine when the body does not move optimally through a golf swing.

Too Much Exercise or Sports

Too much of a good thing can be bad for you as well. Water or oxygen, both of which are vital for life to exist, if consumed in excess can be detrimental for health. Same applies to physical activity.

Case: Resolution—Get Fit!

A few years ago, a thirty-five-year-old senior executive working for a multinational company (MNC) felt tired all the time and had severe back pain. The executive had been a very energetic person, but now he slept through important meetings and was not too productive at work.

When he came to me, the diagnosis was simple: He was suffering from 'overtraining syndrome'. This is a collection of symptoms and behaviours that occur in individuals after repeated strenuous training sessions, with inadequate rest to allow for proper muscle recovery.

On 1 January 2009, the executive had made a new year's resolution to start going to the gym regularly. He started with enthusiasm. He worked out on the treadmill, the cross trainer or the stationary bike every day for more than 45 minutes. He used the weight machines for more than 2 hours each day. He attended as many group classes as possible: power yoga, spinning, core stability—the works. He ate a well-balanced nutritious diet. He stopped eating junk food. The first two months showed a lot of improvement. He felt more energetic at work and was still able to enjoy late-night parties. His wife was impressed by the reducing waistline (from 36 inches to 32 inches).

In March/April, though, he got a bit disappointed: He was fitter than what he was in January, but it was becoming difficult to keep up with the fitness regime. He still partied till late and was punctual at early-morning gym sessions. Most nights, he was sleeping for fewer than 5 hours.

By July/August, the executive's fitness curve was swinging the other way: there was actually deterioration. He could no longer lift as much or do as many repetitions. He didn't last long on the treadmill or the stationary bike. He felt tired all the time. He fell ill often. His wife became concerned. They went to the family doctor. A detailed examination showed that his haemoglobin levels were slightly below normal. Only on their second meeting did the couple mention the executive's new year's resolution. The doctor referred him to a sports medicine expert. And that's where I came in.

Weekend Warrior

Some of you would try to compensate for a very inactive sedentary lifestyle by being overly active during the weekends. If your exercise or sports session ends up being very intense after a week-long sitting, there is a good chance you'll hurt yourself.

Dr William Andrews explains the 'weekend warrior syndrome' really well. 'People who are infrequently excessively active, are at a higher chance of hurting their lower backs.'

Solution

As Mahatma Gandhi has said, 'It is health that is real wealth and not the pieces of gold and silver.' There isn't too much of a correlation between nations winning medals and fitness, e.g., the US, Australia or China.

Participation in sports shouldn't be limited with the goal to win, but to embrace it for life. This needs to start from school, carried on in college and then encouraged in the corporate world.

To maintain good health, thirty to 45 minutes of moderate to vigorous, structured and unstructured physical activity per day is prescribed, but that alone is not ample to fix this problem. Physical activity throughout the day is more important.

Sleeping

On an average, we human beings sleep one-third of our lives. If your posture during sleep is not proper, it is definitely going to ruin your back. Your pillow and mattress needs to be sorted. Also, there is a very good reason that we sleep every night. We need to recover from the hectic day and be fresh for the next one to come. So, if you haven't slept well, it's going to add to your woes.

Solution

Pain can lead to disturbed sleep which in turn causes pain as you feel fatigued throughout the day. This goes on like a vicious circle. Both sleep and pain need to be addressed to break this cycle. Start by sleeping at least for 8 hours.

Living with Pain

> It's all very simple. But maybe because it's so simple, it's also hard.
>
> —Natsuki Takaya, manga comic author

For most people with back pain, the interventions that can be offered in primary care are the only ones that they need.

The physician's attitude and ability to listen to and express empathy with the patient are needed in order to arrive at a mutual understanding concerning treatment strategies. This is also crucial to the future course of back pain and compliance with treatment advice.[22]

Be Better Informed

This is the main focus of the book—to ensure that you are better informed. It is in your best interest. You have to be the one in control and it can only come from being better informed.

Patients often tend to classify their pain as a catastrophe. Misconceptions about the cause of pain and how to appropriately manage it need to be clarified, which is what I have attempted.

Case: Roger Hobbes (name changed), thirty-seven years old

A thirty-seven-year-old former paratrooper from the British Army came to us with severe back pain. He told us that he used to be very active, even in his mid-twenties. He had done over a hundred parachute jumps and put his body through hell. He was now reaping the 'benefits' of what he had sowed. His back pain had begun hampering his daily activities. It was good to see that he was seeing the positive side of it and taking his own condition lightly, but more importantly, he understood that there was no magic pill for pain. He understood that he would have to put in a lot of hard work to undo the mess he was in. He was ready to do it.

Keep Pushing Yourself

To get optimal results from the activities and exercises I have suggested in this book, it is important to keep pushing your comfort zone just that little bit more. Initially, let the pain guide you. If any activity increases the pain, slow down, drop back. Take a break. Then, over the next two–three days, work a little harder at it. Once your pain is more or less manageable, you need to start pushing yourself a little bit more.

Going to the Right Place, Doing the Wrong Things

I recently met a runner during my morning run. He had an anterior cruciate ligament injury in his knee a year ago. He is a regular at a state-of-the-art gym, where he only concentrates on his upper body. He has been told not to work his lower body because of the injury. Even though he is going to the right place, he's simply not doing the right thing. He has been misinformed, which has made him fearful about even going close to the correct strength-training machines.

Rather than blaming everyone else, it becomes his responsibility to find out what works in a condition like his. If the knee is bothering him, he should make an effort to find out what will help improve it.

Don't Avoid Fear

Physical pain leads to psychological pain, which further causes more physical pain, and so a vicious cycle is set into motion. Apprehension of pain makes us avoid doing activities we think will possibly bring on the pain. Encourage yourself to take responsibility.

It is a misconception that activity will make your condition worse. Think a little harder—wouldn't you get weaker if you don't move?

Case: Saloni Mathur (name changed), sixty-seven years old

A sixty-seven-year-old woman suddenly developed a sharp shooting pain down her left leg four months ago. She was rushed to the hospital, where the surgeon advised her to immediately undergo surgery, which she did. Post-surgery, her pain disappeared. She was happy but dreaded having that kind of pain ever again.

The doctor told her to take time off from other activities like walking, which she actually liked doing. She readily agreed and followed the doctor's instructions. Her son happens to be my patient. He told her to start moving again and reclaim her life. He also brought her to me. On examination, I found her to be in a good state of health. I advised her to get on an exercise programme, at first under supervision and then carry on with her life. She was excited about what I had said.

The next day, she broke down in front of the therapist who was taking her session. She told him that her surgeon had yelled at her for seeking help with rehabilitation. He had told her that her condition would worsen again. I didn't push my luck as the surgeon had managed to do something that was very difficult to tackle.

I happened to meet her son a few days later and told him about the damage that surgeon had done. I had only given her hope, but he had 'saved' her from pain. She didn't realize that he had destroyed her life. I told her son that I needed a few sessions just to talk to her, because in her eyes the surgeon was no less than god! Sadly, she did not carry on with her rehabilitation.

In 1960, the then US president John F. Kennedy had written an article in *Sports Illustrated*.[23] He stated:

> For physical fitness is not only one of the most important keys to a healthy body; it is the basis of dynamic and creative intellectual activity. The relationship between the soundness of the body and the activities of the mind is subtle and complex. Much is not yet understood. But we do know what the Greeks knew: that intelligence and skill can only function at the peak of their capacity when the body is healthy and strong; that hardy spirits and tough minds usually inhabit sound bodies.

It might come as a surprise that JFK had such passion for keeping the general population fit. But what you definitely didn't know was that the same year, during his presidential campaign,[24] he was followed everywhere by an aide who carried a bag of 'medical support' because he suffered from severe back pain. He was diagnosed with a degenerative disc disease of the lumbar spine. X-rays from the early 1950s showed a compression fracture of the fifth lumbar vertebrae, for which he had to undergo high-risk back pain surgery.

His back pain didn't improve much after the surgery. He had difficulty bending even slightly forward or backwards. Turning over in bed or sitting down in a chair only made it worse.

He had a first-hand experience with regular exercise therapy with an orthopaedic surgeon (unlike most today) that led to the easing of back spasms and increased his mobility.

Even as a kid, he was frequently ill and suffered from severe fatigue and low weight. He had all the reasons to not do anything and just give up because the experts had said so. Like you, most don't know what an exceptional character JFK was. I need you to be the same.

I had a similar experience with a former health minister of the UK, who had consulted me for her lower back pain. On being told that she should pay more attention to her back, she told me that she had far more important things on her mind that needed addressing than just her back pain. She was talking about the state of National Health Service and how much work needed to be done. That didn't mean she had to ignore the pain; she just had to address it appropriately. She had appropriate bags, did her walks and practised strengthening therapy. Even though her pain persisted, she learnt to live with it.

Miscommunication and Its Effects

Doctors can be reckless with what they say. You need to be aware of which part of their advice to follow, and which to ignore. If it's been a ten-minute consultation and the doctor has said ten positive things, but mentioned in passing the one rare side effect, you would only remember that side effect and it would keep playing on your mind, probably forever.

Think of it differently. You have been with your girlfriend for five years and she is just the most amazing woman. She loves you and takes care of you. One day, while watching the movie *Top Gun*, she comments that 'she finds Tom Cruise cute'. And she never mentions it again. From that day onwards, you start hating Tom Cruise even though *Top Gun* was your favourite film up till that point. You find reasons to avoid going for his films with your girlfriend. There is also a very good chance that 10 per cent of your fights or arguments start at the mention of movies, leave alone Tom Cruise's name.

Case: Kamla Rathore (name changed), sixty-five years old

A sixty-five-year-old woman had been operated sixteen years ago for a disc bulge in her lower back. She was completely pain-free since the surgery. Right after the surgery, the surgeon had told her that her back would be fine for fifteen years. At the end of that duration, she was now terrified that her severe back pain would return. In this case, the surgeon, despite good intentions, had made an error in communication. He made a far-sighted prediction, and might not have realized that the patient would take it so seriously and remember it for that long. This patient wasn't paying attention to the great news that she would be pain-free for fifteen years, but was focusing on the fact that after fifteen years her pain might return. On visiting the doctor recently, he told her she would be fine for another five years. However, by now, she had started feeling the pain.

Placebo Effect

If you come in for treatment with a mindset of not getting better, no one can help you. But when you walk in the door with some conviction, there is a good chance you'll improve. It also helps if you have a smile on your face.

There is evidence to back this statement.

According to the conventional healthcare industry, the placebo effect is useless. Would you mind not being in pain if a sweet homeopathic pill worked for you even though most scientists think that the positive effects of homeopathy are totally placebo? If they don't understand or practise a particular treatment modality and it works, they usually put it under this umbrella.[25]

According to studies, the 'placebo' effect is strongest for the kind, hopeful and straightforward.[26] People in whom 'placebo' has no effect tend to have brains that shrink sooner with ageing.[27] This highlights the fact that it helps to have faith, and this is coming from a non-believer. It possibly is no miracle when a sufferer gets better by a mere touch of a god-man. It's actually his own faith that is healing him. Is it that we don't yet understand 'placebo' and our definition is simply flawed?

There is also evidence to show that exercise plays an important role in preventing the brain from shrinking.[28] In any case, if you play and are physically active, you will not only have a higher pain threshold but will also be smarter (have a sharper brain).

Even ten years ago, 'exercise' was not talked about in medical journals, leave alone being taught at medical colleges. Tons of research is now coming out in favour of exercise and sports. This is happening even though there is no major funding backing the research like the kind any pharmaceutical company normally provides. It's probably because they don't understand a particular 'solution' or it doesn't suit their business model. Why would they promote something that works if it's in direct competition?

Let me explain this with the help of an example. I had been invited to speak at the Second Interventional Pain Conference at AIIMS. One of the senior speakers said that acupuncture is useless as it only has a placebo effect. I pity experts like this. They suffer from a 'since-I-don't-know-it-must-be-rubbish syndrome'. This is not in the best interest of the patient.

Dr Harsh Mahajan, one of India's most respected radiologists and a pioneer in the field of MRI, who was awarded Padma Shri in 2002, narrated a very interesting story to me. One of his close relatives had severe lower back pain and had been to all specialists without any results. Dr Mahajan himself took him to a place that his scientific and medical brain was not ready to accept, but it was out of desperation. There, some sticks were placed on the back and a manoeuvre was done. It somehow worked like magic and the pain disappeared. Dr Mahajan couldn't believe what he had witnessed. Dr Mahajan is a specialist who looks for evidence to determine the cause of pathology. Maybe this only worked for one in twenty or more, but it did work when medical science had given up. There must have been something that worked, maybe something we need to understand. It possibly was spinal manipulation that has been practised in schools in the US and the UK since the 1870s. For instance, it took the medical fraternity three centuries to realize that ether had medical qualities and it could be used for anaesthesia during surgery. Till then, it was simply quackery.

It is simply a myth[29] that there is possibly something wrong with placebo responders. Under appropriate circumstances, any person can become a placebo responder.[30] Fascinatingly, the placebo effect is not limited to non-conventional medicine.

It also brings us to the point that people who exercise regularly, but with a grim face, won't benefit from it. So paste a smile on your face, maybe even laugh and get on with it.

Laughing Clubs

Several parks now have laughing clubs. The act of laughing has been shown to release endorphins, the feel-good hormones that are released during and after exercising. This helps in increasing the pain threshold[31] and also strengthens social bonding.[32]

I propose having laughing clubs everywhere for people suffering from pain. My grumpy colleagues would now probably assume that I've gone looney!

Power of Hugs

Touch is very powerful. Relationships and company are equally important. A Harvard study done over seventy-five years concluded that good relationships keep us healthier and happier, not exercise or nutrition.[33]

I was recently asked if 'hugs' had any musculoskeletal benefits. So I shall only focus on that one treatment modality here. A recent study shows that a good hug needs to be a minimum of 20 seconds to have an effect. A hug helps release 'oxytocin', a hormone secreted by the posterior lobe of the pituitary gland. It is a pea-sized structure at the base of the brain, which calms your nervous system down and boosts positive emotions. It lowers your anxiety and increases happiness. So it's not surprising that hugs can actually reduce pain.

My medical colleagues who talk about 'evidence-based medicine' might contradict me completely. They choose to not believe, without researching about the topic.

I must admit up front that I am an atheist. All I am interested in is helping people get better. Since I mainly focus on pain, I want them to be free of pain for as long as they live. At the same time, I want them to be physically active. So it's about 'miling and smiling' for life. So if I think voodoo would work, I just might give it a shot before saying that it won't work.

Back to 'hugs' and my first experience. I was in the fourth year of my medical college, in OBG (obstetrics and gynaecology) rotation, when I first experienced its effect. An expectant father was standing outside the operation theatre, waiting for his wife who was in labour. He was really concerned because this was their seventh baby. I didn't know how I could help him despite wanting to. I let him hug me. He just cried. But he felt a lot better, he said. All turned out to be fine. It wasn't the hug that made the labour go well, but it reduced his stress immensely. It helped him calm down. Being stressed wasn't going to solve anything anyway.

For a very long time, even after this incident, I had hug-phobia. It's only recently that I have become comfortable with it.

Isn't it fun to note that people in all religions say that when you pray, pray with all your heart, only then will your prayers be addressed? The same holds true for hugs, I feel. So, when you hug someone the next time, don't hold back.

The Thinking Sufferer

I need you to be like a surfer who has to tackle all kinds of waves. Plan A is just not good enough because it will fail. It's like Murphy's Law: Whatever can go wrong, will go wrong. Be prepared for it. If things aren't going as per plan, be prepared to change accordingly. You need to be strong and flexible in mind and body. If you stiffen up in either, it's going to hurt a lot more.

Even with the best of rehabilitation programmes, the intensity of pain goes up and down like a stock market graph. As long as the graph is generally going in the right direction, don't worry about a few dips or surges here and there. If for no rhyme or reason, the pain disappears one day, don't get super-excited. You've been doing something right. Keep at it. But don't get ahead of yourself. Keep it slow and steady. On the flip side, if for no reason the pain worsens one morning, don't get worked up. Getting stressed will not help you. Focus on breathing. Think about your posture.

Let me take the analogy of stock markets a bit further. When you invest in stocks, you can't and shouldn't be scrutinizing them every minute of every hour of every day of every month for the whole year. There are 5,25,600 minutes in a year if it's not a leap year. You should look at the bigger picture.

If there are too many surges in pain, however, you do need to plan differently or change your approach. What is definitely not worth it is the cafeteria approach to medical advice. If you have asked a doctor or two, you are doing well. As mentioned earlier, please don't fall for ill-informed discouraging advice. You are well equipped by now to know what is right for you. You do need to be active, and conservative management of your back pain is the way to go.

If things have not gone according to your plan, you simply need to apply the advice already given to you. Logical thinking with a cool head is all that is needed.

If you haven't watched *Sherlock Holmes: A Game of Shadows*, I recommend you do so. In the film, Holmes, before picking a fight with anyone, runs through the motion of actions in his head. His last fight with his adversary, Professor Moriarty, turns out to be a great lesson. More than a fight, it is about the anticipation of the attack and the counter-attack. There is much to be learnt from this scene. Holmes uses a technique called 'visualization', also called guided imagery or mental rehearsal. Prior to this scene, Moriarty manages to injure Holmes's right shoulder. After a detailed prediction of moves from him and counter-moves from Moriarty, Holmes deduces that Moriarty would most likely kill him by focusing his deadly punches and kicks on his injured right shoulder. That's when Holmes decides to approach the situation differently.

You too need to become smart and analytical, and not just a strong person bulldozing through life. You need to visualize every possible scenario and take decisions accordingly. For different situations, you should have different plans in place. I want you to be more aware human beings; for this, you need to be able to listen to your body and also be attuned to your surroundings.

I want you to be a Sherlock Holmes, not necessarily in trying to find the diagnosis but in trying to understand what triggered the pain and what had worked for you in the past.

Summary: Smile More

To sum it all up, always remind yourself that we were born to die. It's entirely up to us how we spend our time between these two incidents that, in bigger schemes of things, don't matter at all. Fair enough, that pain is inevitable as it is part of life, but then suffering is optional.

Have you ever noticed that the skeleton is always smiling but courtesy the society, there is a preconceived notion that skeletons are scary. The next time you look at the skull, check out that smile. Somehow, as soon as we are born we start crying. Throughout our lives we end up mastering that frown. We need to smile more. It'll help us calm down.

The cadavers in the dissection rooms did teach us, the doctors, an immense lot. Yet, things are slightly different when we are alive. Besides moving, we are also thinking beings. Along with understanding this, we need to first understand what is healthy and normal, before we aspire to get our clients there. Let go of those preconceived notions, whether they are about a skeleton being scary or the back being the cause of pain. There are known cases of people having a heart attack simply by looking at a skull in the dark because of how it has been portrayed in films and books. It is a question of changing your outlook. Let's press the reset button.

We, as a society, are looking for a change, we need to be the solution, rather than contribute to the problem at hand. Let's all start with ourselves, spread the good habits amongst our immediate friends and family, even if it's only one.

Don't resist. Let go.
Let's get moving, now!
Keep miling and smiling.

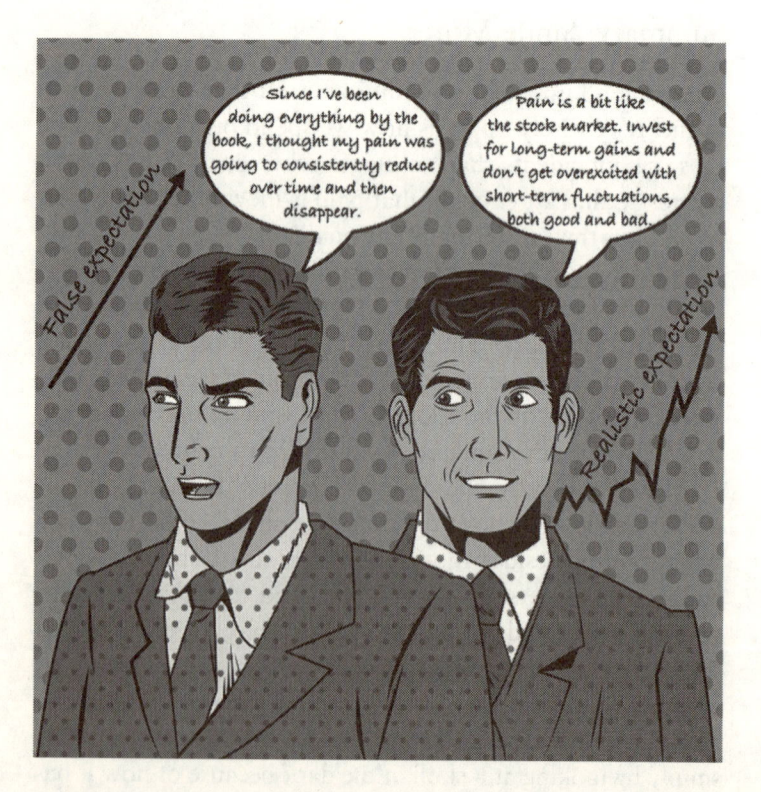

ACKNOWLEDGEMENTS

If I have seen further it is by standing on the shoulders of giants.
—Isaac Newton

All my teachers, throughout the years, have been these giants for me. Thanks a million miles to all of you.

Thank you Ira Leinonen and Jamie Skelly for showing me how overrated educational degrees are. I learnt more about movement, strength training and rehabilitation from you two than anyone else.

Below are names of other professional colleagues whom I very highly respect in medical fraternity. They have knowingly or unknowingly contributed towards my learnings of the subject.

Prof. Steven N. Blair, Dr Karim Khan, Dr P.S. Chandran, Prof. Stuart McGill, Prof. Timothy Noakes, Peter Halen, Dr B.K. Singh, Dr B.K. Rao, Dr Harsh Mahajan, Dr Raju Eshwaran, Dr Pankaj Surange, Dr Thomas Kishen, Dr Sanjay Dhawan, and my good friends, Dr Vikram Kumar and Dr Anurag Mishra.

'If you want to master something, teach it.' This old adage helped me immensely while I trained my team from scratch rather than expecting them to know it all from before. Most of the times, there was a lot of unlearning for them to do. Teaching them the basics made me question the obvious again and again, which otherwise is overlooked. All my team members have directly or indirectly contributed to this book. They also made me realize that I had become more of a student of pain for life rather than a master.

Below are names of colleagues, in no particular order, for all their contributions. If I have forgotten anyone, I apologize. You know who you are. I sincerely appreciate all your contributions:

Vishwanathan Sridharan, Kunal Vashist, Karishma Rathore, Ritika Chawla, Gagandeep Kaur, Sonam Taneja, Sunil Dahiya, Kishan Pesswani, Neha Kumar, Nimrat Kaur, Sumanth Kumar, Anuvrat Singh, Shibani James, Ishan Arora, Samridhi Saxena, Anika Kaur, Dipali Dhamija, Sumit Arora, Vidhushi Wadehra, Munesh Kumar, Nandlal Pathak, Garima Chawla, Anjeline Dhaka, Krishna Prem, Debapriya Kapoor, Preeti Ashok, Sahrika Sankla, Anita Mathews, Princey, Magesh Kumar, Shahbaz Nawaz, Sudeep Gurang and Kieran Lowe.

Thank you Supreet J. Bargi for doing the photoshoot at such a short notice for the exercises. Thank you Ritika Chawla for agreeing to model, and Karishma Rathore, Vishwanathan Sridharan, Kunal Vashist and Gagandeep Kaur for all the logistics involved in making it happen. Thank you Catherine Withers for helping with editing my random thoughts and giving them shape. Thank you Saloni Mital for making sense out of it all. A special thanks to Shahnaz Siganporia for proposing this idea and helping me build the skeletal structure.

My brats Viren and Harsheath showed me that pain is simply fun. Befriend it and get on with life. Apologies to you both and your mom and my wife, Nidhi, for spending a lot of time on this 'Taj Mahal of a book', which should have come out three years ago.

I get too emotionally involved with my patients' condition. At times it drains me, particularly when their pain doesn't improve. Thank you so much, Dad, for encouraging me to stay the way I've always been because, as you say, that's what makes me unique. My mother has been my rock through thick and thin, and I can't thank her enough.

NOTES

Prologue: Why Me?

1. O'Leary, T.J., M.G. Morris, J. Collett, and K. Howells, 'Central and peripheral fatigue following non-exhaustive and exhaustive exercise of disparate metabolic demands', *Scandinavian Journal of Medicine and Science in Sports*, 2015.
2. Noakes, Timothy, *Challenging Beliefs: Memoirs of a Career*, Penguin Random House South Africa, 2012.
3. La Ultra—The High, www.laultra.in.

1. Why You Need This Book

1. Murray, C.J., T. Vos, R. Lozano, et al., 'Disability-adjusted life years (DALYs) for 291 diseases and injuries in 21 regions, 1990–2010: A systematic analysis for the Global Burden of Disease Study 2010', *Lancet*, Vol. 380, No. 9859, 2012, pp.2197–2223.
2. Jonsson, Egon, *Back Pain, Next Pain*, (translated by Ron Gustafson), 2000, http://www.sbu.se/upload/Publikationer/Content0/1/back_neckpain_2000/backpainslut.pdf.
3. Ibid.
4. Buddhist Sangha of South Jersey, http://buddhistsangha.tripod.com/noblepath2.htm.

5. Allan D.B. and G. Waddell, 'An historical perspective on low back pain and disability', *Acta Orthopaedica Scandinavica*, 1989, http://dx.doi.org/10.3109/17453678909153916.
6. Pausanias, *Description of Greece* (translated by Jones, W.H.S.), http://www.theoi.com/Ther/DrakainaPoine. Html.
7. Allan, D.B. and Waddell G., 'An historical perspective on low back pain and disability', *Acta Orthopaedica Scandinavica*, 1989, http://dx.doi.org/10.3109/17453678909153916.
8. Keele, K.D., *Anatomies of Pain*, Oxford: Blakewell Scientific Publications, 1957.
9. 'Ancient Egyptian Herbalism', HubPages, http://chermarie.hubpages.com/hub/AncientEgyptianHerbalism.
10. Lallanilla, Marc, 'A brief history of Pain', ABC News, 2005, http://abcnews.go.com/Health/PainManagement/story?id=731553&page=1#.UX1hwCv89gs.
11. Ibid.
12. Allan, D.B. and G. Waddell, 'An historical perspective on low back pain and disability', *Acta Orthopaedica Scandinavica*, 1989, http://dx.doi.org/10.3109/17453678909153916.
13. Erichsen, J.E., *On Concussion of the Spine: Nervous Shock and Other Obscure Injuries to the Nervous System in Their Clinical and Medico-Legal Aspects*, London: Walton & Maberly, 1866.
14. Paul, Barash G., et al, *Clinical Anesthesia*, Philadelphia: Lippincott Williams and Wilkins, 2013.
15. 'Anesthesia and Queen Victoria', Department of Epidemiology, University of California, Los Angeles, http://www.ph.ucla.edu/epi/snow/victoria.html.
16. Lallanilla, Marc, 'A Brief History of Pain', ABC News, 2005, http://abcnews.go.com/Health/PainManagement/story?id=731553&page=1#.UX1hwCv89gs.
17. Allan, D.B. and G. Waddell, 'An historical perspective on low back pain and disability', *Acta Orthopaedica Scandinavica*, 1989, http://dx.doi.org/10.3109/17453678909153916.
18. Walser, H.H., 'Ruckenschmerzen in der Geschichte der Medizin', J. Praxis, 1969.

19. MacDonald, R.S., *Back Pain: Classification of Syndromes*, Manchester: Manchester University Press, 1990.
20. Allan, D.B. and G. Waddell, 'An historical perspective on low back pain and disability', *Acta Orthopaedica Scandinavica*, 1989, http://dx.doi.org/10.3109/17453678909153916.

2. Getting to Know Yourself

1. Ornish, Dean, 'Ted Talk: Your genes are not your fate', March 2008, http://www.ted.com/talks/dean_ornish_says_your_genes_are_not_your_fate?language=en.
2. Wolpert, Daniel, 'Ted Talk: The Real Reasons for Brains', July 2011, https://www.ted.com/talks/daniel_wolpert_the_real_reason_for_brains?language=en.
3. Butler, David, 'Treating pain using the Brain', YouTube, https://www.youtube.com/watch?v=4ABAS3tkkuE.
4. Vehicle frame, Wikipedia, https://en.wikipedia.org/wiki/Vehicle_frame.
5. Finando, Donna, Trigger Point Self-Care Manual: For Pain-Free Movement, Simon & Schuster, 2005.
6. Ibid.
7. Panjabi, M.M., 'The stabilizing system of the spine, Part I: Function, dysfunction, adaptation, and enhancement', Journal of Spinal Disorders, Vol.5, No.4, 1992, pp.383–9.
8. Liebenson, Craig, 'Spinal Stabilization', Journal of Bodywork and Movement Therapy, Vol.8, 2004, pp.199–210.
9. McGill, S. M., Resource Manual for Guidelines for Exercise Testing and Prescription, Philadelphia, Williams and Wilkins, 1998.
10. Nicholls, Carolyn, The Posture Workbook, United Kingdom: D&B Publishing, 2012.

3. What You Should Do When You Have Back Pain

1. Noakes, Timothy, *Challenging Beliefs: Memoirs of a Career,* Penguin Random House South Africa, 2012.

2. Hutson, Michael, *Textbook of Musculoskeletal Medicine*, Oxford: Oxford University Press, 2006.
3. Ibid.
4. 'The Australian Physiotherapy Association: Tests, treatments and procedures physiotherapists and consumers should question', Choosing Wisely Australia, http://www.choosingwisely.org.au/recommendations/apa.
5. Charlie Gregory, contributor, UK.
6. 'The Society of Hospital Pharmacists of Australia: Treatments pharmacists and consumers should question, Choosing Wisely Australia', http://www.choosingwisely.org.au/recommendations/shpa.
7. Ibid.

4. Tests and Investigations

1. Hutson, Michael, Oxford Textbook of Musculoskeletal Medicine, Oxford: Oxford University Press, 2015.
2. 'The Australian Physiotherapy Association: Tests, treatments and procedures physiotherapists and consumers should question', Choosing Wisely Australia, www.choosingwisely.org.au/recommendations/apa#collapse-1; also, developed by the Royal Australian and New Zealand College of Radiologists.
3. Nachemson, Alf, 'Low-back pain: Are Orthopedic surgeons missing the boat?', Acta Orthop Scand, Vol.9, No.1, 1994, pp.1–2.
4. Hutson, Michael, *Textbook of Musculoskeletal Medicine*, Oxford: Oxford University Press, 2006.
5. 'Low back pain in adults: Early management', NICE Clinical Guidelines, 27 May 2009, www.nice.org.uk/guidance/cg88/resources/low-back-pain-in-adultsearly-management-975695607493.
6. O'Sullivan K. and P. O'Sullivan, 'The ineffectiveness of paracetamol for spinal pain provides opportunities to

better manage low back pain', British Journal of Sports Medicine, Vol.50, No.4, 2016, pp.197–8.

7. 'Low back pain in adults: Early management', NICE Clinical Guidelines, 27 May 2009, www.nice.org.uk/guidance/cg88/resources/low-back-pain-in-adultsearly-management-975695607493.

8. Ibid.

9. Sinaiko, Anna, Meredith B. Rosenthal, 'Examining A Health Care Price Transparency Tool: Who Uses It And How They Shop For Care', *Health Affairs*, Vol.35, No.4, April 2016, pp. 662–670.

10. Jarvik J.J., W. Hollingworth, P. Heagerty, D.R. Haynor, R.A. Deyo, 'The Longitudinal Assessment of Imaging and Disability of the Back (LAIDBack) Study: Baseline Data', The Spine Journal, Vol. 30, No. 13, May 2001, pp.1541–1548; see also, McCullough B.J., G.R. Johnson, B.I. Martin, J.G. Jarvik, 'Lumbar MR imaging and reporting epidemiology: Do epidemiologic data in reports affect clinical management?', *Radiology*, Vol.262, No.3, March 2012, pp.941–6.

11. Morita M., A. Miyauchi, S. Okuda, T. Oda and M. Iwasaki, 'Comparison between MRI and myelography in lumbar spinal canal stenosis for the decision of levels of decompression surgery', Journal of Spinal Disorders, Vol.24, No.1, 2011, pp.31–6.

12. Bartynski W.S., L. Lin, 'Lumbar root compression in the lateral recess: MR imaging, conventional myelography, and CT myelography comparison with surgical confirmation', American Journal of Neuroradiology, Vol.24, 2003, pp.348–360.

13. Heidari P., F. Farahbakhsh, M. Rostami, P. Noormohammadpour and R. Kordi, 'The Role of Ultrasound in Diagnosis of the Causes of Low Back Pain: A Review of the Literature', *Asian Journal of Sports Medicine*, Vol.6, No.1, March 2015.

5. Common Diagnosis: Causes of Back Pain

1. Jonsson, Egon, *Back Pain, Next Pain*, (translated by Ron Gustafson), 2000, http://www.sbu.se/upload/Publikationer/Content0/1/back_neckpain_2000/backpainslut.pdf.
2. Jarvik J.J., W. Hollingworth, P. Heagerty, D.R. Haynor, R.A. Deyo, 'The Longitudinal Assessment of Imaging and Disability of the Back (LAIDBack) Study: Baseline Data', The Spine Journal, Vol. 30, No. 13, May 2001, pp.1541–1548.
3. Finando, Donna, Trigger Point Self-Care Manual: For Pain-Free Movement, Simon & Schuster, 2005.
4. Wadell, G., 'Understanding and management of low back pain', Acta Orthop Scand, Vol.60, No.234, 1989, pp.1–23. For history of back pain, this paper has been used extensively as it's rich in information. But the interpretations are the author's.
5. Strauss W.L., A.J.E. Cave, 'Pathology and the posture of Neanderthal man', Quarterly Review of Biology, Vol.32, 1957, pp.348–363.
6. Blumberg, B.S., L. Sokoloff, 'Coalescence of caudal vertebrae in the giant dinosaur Diplodocus', *Arthritis and Rheumatology*, Vol.4, 1961, pp.592–601.
7. Bourke, J.B, 'The Palaeopathology of the vertebral body in Ancient Egypt and Nubia', Medical History, Vol.15, No.4,1971, pp.363–375; see also, McKem, W.,T.D. Stewart, 'Archeology: Skeletal age changes in young American males', American Anthropologist, Vol.50, No.5, 1958, pp.982; and also, Lawrence, J.S., J.M. Bremmer, F. Bier, 'Osteo-arthrosis prevalence in the population and relationship between symptoms and x-ray changes', *Annals of the Rheumatic Diseases*, Vol.25, No.1, 1966, pp.1–24.
8. Bourke, J.B., 'The Palaeopathology of the vertebral column in Ancient Egypt and Nubia', Medical History, Vol.15, No.4, 1971, pp.363-375; see also, Promiska, E., 'The role of palaeopathology in modern medicine', Mater Med Pol, Vol.18. No.4, 1986, pp.211–7.

9. Wadell, G., 'Understanding and management of low back pain', Acta Orthop Scand, Vol.60, No.234, 1989, pp.1–23. For history of back pain, this paper has been used extensively as it's rich in information. But the interpretations are the author's.

6. Proactively Managing Back Pain

1. Contributor: Physiotherapist Manish Tiwari.
2. Jonsson, Egon, *Back Pain, Next Pain*, (translated by Ron Gustafson), 2000, http://www.sbu.se/upload/Publikationer/Content0/1/back_neckpain_2000/backpainslut.pdf.
3. McGill, Stuart, Ultimate Back Fitness and Performance, 2004.
4. McGill, S., J. Seguin, and J. Bennett, 'Passive stiffness of the lumbar torso in flexion, extension, lateral bending, and axial rotation: Effect of belt wearing and breath holding', *Spine Journal*, Vol.19, No.6, 1994, pp.696–704.
5. O'Sullivan K. and P. O'Sullivan, 'The ineffectiveness of paracetamol for spinal pain provides opportunities to better manage low back pain', British Journal of Sports Medicine, Vol.50, No.4, 2016, pp.197–8.
6. Derry, S., R.A. Moore, H. Gaskell, M. McIntyre and P.J. Wiffen, 'Topical NSAIDS for Acute Musculoskeletal Pain in Adults', Cochrane Database of Systematic Reviews, 2015.
7. 'Siesta', http://en.wikipedia.org/wiki/Siesta.
8. McGill, Stuart, Ultimate Back Fitness and Performance, 2004.

7. The Three Musketeers: Foot (and Ankle), Knee and Hip (FKH)

1. Contributors: Ritika Chawla, Karishma Rathore, J.S.Viswanathan, Garima Chawla. All physiotherapists at Back 2 Fitness clinic.
2. 'The global burden of low back pain: Estimates from the Global Burden of Disease 2010 study', Annals of

the Rheumatic Diseases, 2014, http://ard.bmj.com/content/73/6/968.full.
3. Ibid.
4. Ibid.
5. Liu, S. H. and W.J. Jason, 'Lateral ankle sprains and instability problems', *Clinics in Sports Medicine*, Vol.13, No.4, 1994, pp.793–809.
6. McCormack, R.G. and M.R. Hutchinson, 'Time to be honest regarding outcomes of ACL reconstructions', *British Journal of Sports Medicine*, Vol.50, No.19, 2016, pp.1167–8.
7. Ardern, C.L., N.F. Taylor, J.A. Feller, et al, 'Fifty-five per cent return to competitive sport following anterior cruciate ligament reconstruction surgery: An updated systematic review and meta-analysis including aspects of physical functioning and contextual factors', *British Journal of Sports Medicine*, Vol.48, No.21, 2014, pp.1543–52; see also, Waldén, M., M. Hagglund, H. Magnusson, et al, 'ACL injuries in men's professional football: A 15-year prospective study on time trends and return-to-play rates reveals only 65% of players still play at the top level 3 years after ACL rupture', *British Journal of Sports Med*, Vol.50, No.12, 2016, pp.744–50; and also, Wiggins, A.J., R.K. Grandhi, D.K. Schneider, et al, 'Risk of secondary injury in younger athletes after anterior cruciate ligament reconstruction: a systematic review and metaanalysis', *American Journal of Sports Medicine*, Vol.44, No.7, 2016, pp.1861–76.
8. Waldén, M., M.Hagglund, H.Magnusson, et al, 'ACL injuries in men's professional football: A 15-year prospective study on time trends and return-to-play rates reveals only 65% of players still play at the top level 3 years after ACL rupture', *British Journal of Sports Med*, Vol.50, No.12, 2016, pp.744–50.
9. McCormack, R.G. and M.R. Hutchinson, 'Time to be honest regarding outcomes of ACL reconstructions',

British Journal of Sports Medicine, Vol.50, No.19, 2016, pp.1167–8.
10. Grindem, H., L. Snyder-Mackler., H. Moksnes, et al, 'Simple decision rules can reduce reinjury risk by 84% after ACL reconstruction, British Journal of Sports Medicine, 2016.
11. Wiggins, A.J., R.K. Grandhi, D.K. Schneider, et al, 'Risk of secondary injury in younger athletes after anterior cruciate ligament reconstruction: a systematic review and metaanalysis', *American Journal of Sports Medicine*, Vol.44, No.7, 2016, pp.1861–76.
12. Grindem, H., L. Snyder-Mackler., H. Moksnes, et al, 'Simple decision rules can reduce reinjury risk by 84% after ACL reconstruction, British Journal of Sports Medicine, 2016.
13. Shelbourne, Don, BJSM Podcast, 27 May 2016, https://soundcloud.com/bmjpodcasts/the-father-of-acceleratedrehabilitation-dr-don-shelbourne-on-history-andmanaging-acl-injuries.
14. Contributors: Physiotherapists Ishan Arora, Shibani James.
15. Contributors: Physiotherapist Neha Kumar and Kunal Vashist.

8. Other Common Aches and Pains

1. Contributors: Physiotherapists Ritika Chawla and Kunal Vashist.
2. Contributor: Dr Anurag Mishra, psychiatrist and psychoanalytical psychotherapist.
3. Gowers, William, 'A Lecture on Lumbago: Its Lessons and Analogues', British Medical Journal, Vol.1, No.2246, 1904, pp.117–121.

9. Pain Is Inevitable, Suffering Is Optional

1. A quote by Lama Surya Das, an American lama in the Tibetan Buddhist tradition. He is a poet, chant master,

spiritual activist and author of many popular works on Buddhism.
2. Dr William Andrews, an authority in unlocking the molecular mechanisms of ageing; president and chief executive officer of Sierra Sciences, a company devoted to finding ways of lengthening telomeres.
3. Jonsson, Egon, *Back Pain, Next Pain*, (translated by Ron Gustafson), 2000, http://www.sbu.se/upload/Publikationer/Content0/1/back_neckpain_2000/backpainslut.pdf.
4. Diamond, Jared, 'The Worst Mistake in the History of the Human Race,' Discover Magazine, 1999, http://discovermagazine.com/1987/may/02-the-worst-mistake-in-the-history-of-the-human-race.
5. Haldane, Andrew, The Pacific, Season 1, Episode 7, 'Peleliu Hills'.
6. Contributors: Physiotherapists Kavita and Kunal Vashist.
7. 'Physical activity and exercise during pregnancy and the postpartum period', Committee Opinion No. 650, The American College of Obstetricians and Gynecologists, 2015, http://www.acog.org/Resources-And-Publications/Committee-Opinions/Committee-on-Obstetric-Practice/Physical-Activity-and-Exercise-During-Pregnancy-and-the-Postpartum-Period.
8. Gupta, Garima and Nupur Nandini, 'Prevalence of low back pain in non-working rural housewives of Kanpur, India', International Journal of Occupational Medicine and Environment Health, Vol.28, No.2, 2015, pp.313–20.
9. Blair, Steven, Paul Thompson, Tim Church, 'Exercise in the Age of Evidence-Based Medicine: A Clinical Update', Medscape, 18 December 2006.
10. Case, Anne and Christina Paxson, 'Parental behavior and child health', Project HOPE—The People-To-People Health Foundation, March/April 2002, pp.167, https://www.princeton.edu/~accase/downloads/Parental_Behavior_and_Child_HealthA.pdf.

11. Cleland, V., et al, 'Parental exercise is associated with Australian children's extracurricular sports participation and cardiorespiratory fitness: A cross-sectional study', International Journal of Behavioral Nutrition and Physical Activity, Vol.2, No.3, 2005.
12. Morris, J.N., J.A. Heady, P.A. Raffle, C.G. Roberts and J.W. Parks, 'Coronary heart-disease and physical activity of work', Lancet, Vol. 265, No. 6795, 1953, pp.1053–57.
13. Gangopadhyay, S. and S.Dev, 'Effect of low back pain on social and professional life of drivers of Kolkata', Work, Vol. 41, 2012, pp.2426–2433.
14. Dr Micklewright, University of Essex, http://www.essex.ac.uk/events/event.aspx?e_id=1670.
15. Steffens, D., et al, 'Prevention of Low Back Pain: A Systematic Review and Meta-analysis', JAMA Internal Medicine, Vol.176, No.2, 2016, pp.199–208.
16. Contributor: Kishan Pesswani, a fitness enthusiast.
17. Hoy D., et al., 'The global burden of low back pain: Estimates from the Global Burden of Disease 2010 study', Annals of Rheumatic Diseases, Vol. 73, No.6, 2014, pp.968–974.
18. Ibid.
19. Ekelund U., et al, 'Does physical activity attenuate, or even eliminate, the detrimental association of sitting time with mortality? A harmonized meta-analysis of data from more than 1 million men and women', Lancet, Vol.388, No.10051, 2016, pp.1302–10.
20. Chauhan, Rajat, 'Are you fit enough to play', Livemint, 2010, http://www.livemint.com/Leisure/bWVum9E6Ggh0DiN9pVQ25L/Are-you-fit-enough-to-play.html.
21. Chauhan, Rajat, 'Golf and back pain' Livemint, 3 August 2009.
22. Jonsson, Egon, *Back Pain, Next Pain*, (translated by Ron Gustafson), 2000, http://www.sbu.se/upload/Publikationer/Content0/1/back_neckpain_2000/backpainslut.pdf.

23. Kennedy, John F., 'The Soft American', *Sports Illustrated*, http://sportsillustrated.cnn.com/vault/article/magazine/MAG1134750/2/index.htm.
24. Eisenbraun, Karen, 'John F Kennedy—A life of back pain and hidden lies', http://www.vacupractor.com/famouspeople/john-f-kennedy-back-pain/.
25. Second Interventional Pain Conference at AIIMS, New Delhi.
26. Healy, Melissa, 'Placebo effect is strongest for the kind, hopeful, straightforward', Los Angeles Times, http://www.latimes.com/health/boostershots/la-heb-placebo-effectpersonality- 20121115,0,1423424.story.
27. Benedetti, Fabrizio, Elisa Carlino and Antonella Pollo, 'How Placebos Change the Patient's Brain', Neuropsychopharmacology, Vol.36, No.1, 2011, http://www.nature.com/npp/journal/v36/n1/full/npp201081a.html.
28. Roberts, Michelle, 'Exercising in your 70s may stop brain shrinkage', BBC News online, 2012, http://www.bbc.co.uk/news/health-20026099.
29. Cohen, Milton C., 'Placebo Theory', *Textbook of Musculoskeletal Medicine*, Oxford: Oxford University Press, 2015.
30. Voudouris, N. J., C.L. Peck, G. Coleman, 'Conditioned response models of placebo phenomena', Pain, Vol.31, No.1, 1989, pp.109–16.
31. Dunbar, R. I. M., et al., 'Social laughter is correlated with an elevated pain threshold', 2012, http://rspb.royalsocietypublishing.org/content/279/1731/1161.full.pdf+html.
32. Cadena, Viviana, 'Let us laugh to ease the pain', *The Journal of Experimental Biology*, 2012, http://jeb.biologists.org/content/215/15/iv.full.
33. 'Good relationships keep us healthier and happier—lessons from a 75-year long Harvard Study', https://t.co/qoCGEfDfml.

SOURCES FOR PHOTOGRAPHS AND ILLUSTRATIONS

- Illustrations on pages xxvi, 17, 50, 78, 92, 104, 157, 200, 212, 284 are by Jemastock.
- Illustrations on pages 24, 27, 30, 32, 33, 34, 40 are by Adimas.
- Photos on pages 110, 119, 121, 122, 123, 124, 125, 126, 127, 128, 129, 130, 131, 132, 134, 135, 136, 137, 138, 139, 140, 141, 142, 160, 162, 164, 166 are by Supreet J. Bargi.
- Photo on page xxiv is by Upslope Productions.